W9-BJB-147

USING THE

FIELDWORK

PERFORMANCE

EVALUATION

FORMS

The Complete Guide

By Karen Atler, MS, OTR

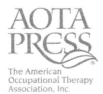

AOTA PRESS

The American
Occupational Therapy
Association, Inc.

Mission Statement
The American Occupational Therapy Association advances the quality, availability, use,
and support of occupational therapy through standard-setting, advocacy, education, and research
on behalf of its members and the public.

AOTA Staff
Joseph C. Isaacs, CAE, Executive Director
Karen C. Carey, CAE, Associate Executive Director, Membership, Marketing, and Communications

Frank E. Gainer, MHS, OTR/L, FAOTA, Education Program Manager

Chris Davis, Managing Editor, AOTA Press
Suzanne Seitz, Production Editor, AOTA Press
Barbara Dickson, Editorial Assistant

Robert A. Sacheli, Manager, Creative Services
Sarah E. Ely, Book Production Coordinator

The American Occupational Therapy Association, Inc.
4720 Montgomery Lane
PO Box 31220
Bethesda, MD 20824-1220
Phone: 301-652-AOTA (2682)
TDD: 800-377-8555
Fax: 301-652-7711
www.aota.org
To order: 1-877-404-AOTA (2682)

© 2003 by The American Occupational Therapy Association, Inc. All rights reserved.
No part of this book may be reproduced in whole or in part by any means without permission.
Printed in the United States of America.

Library of Congress Control Number: 2003106032

ISBN: 1-56900-185-5

Disclaimers
This publication is designed to provide accurate and authoritative information in regard to the subject
matter covered. It is sold or distributed with the understanding that the publisher is not engaged in rendering
legal, accounting, or other professional service. If legal advice or other expert assistance is required, the
services of a competent professional person should be sought.
—*From the Declaration of Principles jointly adopted by the American Bar Association
and a Committee of Publishers and Associations*

It is the objective of The American Occupational Therapy Association to be a forum for free expression and
interchange of ideas. The opinions expressed by the contributors to this work are their own and not necessarily
those of The American Occupational Therapy Association.

Printed by Nittany Valley Offset, State College, PA

Contents

Acknowledgments

The project could not have been completed without the assistance and contribution of many individuals. Their willingness to volunteer their time, efforts, and expertise was invaluable to the completion of this project. My thanks go to each of you!

Contributing Authors

- **Roberta Wimmer, OTR/L,** Academic Fieldwork Coordinator, Pacific University, Forest Grove, OR; Cochair, Fieldwork Evaluation Revision Task Force, 1998–2002
- **Anne G. Fisher, ScD, OTR, FAOTA,** Professor, Colorado State University, Fort Collins

Reviewers

- **Donna M. Costa, MS, OTR/L,** Academic Fieldwork Coordinator, State University of New York at Stony Brook
- **Kathy Splinter-Watkins, MOT, OTR/L,** Level II Academic Fieldwork Coordinator, Eastern Kentucky University, Richmond
- **Patricia Stutz-Tanenbaum, MS, OTR,** Academic Fieldwork Coordinator, Colorado State University, Fort Collins
- **Barbara Borg, MA, OTR,** Assistant Professor, Colorado State University, Fort Collins
- **Frank E. Gainer, MHS, OTR/L, FAOTA,** Education Program Manager, American Occupational Therapy Association, Bethesda, MD

Support Staff

The Colorado State University Occupational Therapy Department provided resources and staff support. Special thanks go to Lynsie MacMasters and Kelly Freidel.

Fieldwork Evaluation Revision Task Force Members

- **Carole W. Dennis, ScD, OTR/L, BCP,** Ithaca College, New York
- **Carole Hays, MA, OTR/L, FAOTA,** Springfield Hospital Center, Sykesville, MD
- **Becky Robler, MEd, OTR,** Pueblo Community College, Pueblo, CO

Additional Supporters of the Project

- **Anne G. Fisher, ScD, OTR, FAOTA,** Professor, Colorado State University, Fort Collins
- **Brenda Merritt, MS, OTR,** doctoral candidate, Colorado State University, Fort Collins
- **Doris Gordon, MS, MPH, OTR, FAOTA,** Former Director of Academic and International Affairs, American Occupational Therapy Association, Bethesda, MD
- Patients at the Springfield Hospital Center in Sykesville, MD
- Academic fieldwork coordinators, fieldwork educators, and students from across the United States who provided input and feedback through reviewing, piloting, or critiquing the evaluation forms throughout the development process.

CHAPTER 1

Overview

The *Fieldwork Performance Evaluation for the Occupational Therapy Student (FWPE/OTS)* and the *Fieldwork Performance Evaluation for the Occupational Therapy Assistant Student (FWPE/OTAS)* were adopted in August 2002 by the American Occupational Therapy Association's (AOTA's) Commission on Education (COE), replacing AOTA's 1987 *Fieldwork Evaluation for the Occupational Therapist* and its 1983 *Fieldwork Evaluation Form for Occupational Therapy Assistant Students.* These new evaluations will help fieldwork educators determine whether students are ready for entry-level practice by assessing whether the objectives of fieldwork have been met. The primary purpose of fieldwork is to develop entry-level occupational therapists and occupational therapy assistants who possess (a) competency to deliver occupational therapy services across practice settings and (b) sound, logical, and ethical clinical reasoning (American Council for Occupational Therapy Education [ACOTE], 1999a, 1999b).

In fall of 1998, the Fieldwork Evaluation Revision Task Force was charged with revising/developing companion documents to measure entry-level competence of occupational therapy and occupational therapy assistant Level II fieldwork students. *Entry-level competence* was defined as the ability to engage in the occupational therapy process rather than perform individual skills. The COE, the task force, and occupational therapy practitioners who responded to surveys wanted the new forms to

- apply across all practice settings,
- focus on occupation-based practice,
- reflect both current and future practice,
- provide feedback to students, and
- be user-friendly to fieldwork educators (i.e., able to be completed in a timely manner).

The fieldwork performance evaluation forms for occupational therapy students and occupational therapy assistant students were created as companion documents that share the same guiding structure: the major steps of the occupational therapy process. Chapter 2 reviews the major documents used to guide the devel-

opment of these forms. These documents highlight not only the key aspects of the occupational therapy process, the necessary knowledge and skills to carry out the process, or both, but also the collaborative nature of the relationship between occupational therapists and occupational therapy assistants during the occupational therapy process.

Rationale and Purpose

The new fieldwork performance evaluation forms were developed because both fieldwork educators and students had commented over the years that the previous evaluations were out of date, no longer reflected current practice, and were not compatible with the expansion of fieldwork sites into emerging community-based practice settings. Two studies (Kirchner, Stone, & Holm, 2001; Stutz-Tanenbaum, Gaffney, Bundy, & Fisher, 1993) clearly supported the expressed concern of fieldwork educators to revise the evaluations. (See chapter 3 for more details.) After a review of education and practice documents and literature regarding fieldwork, clinical reasoning, competency, and measurement, the fieldwork performance evaluation forms were designed with two purposes in mind:

1. to evaluate whether a student's performance meets competency for entry-level practice and
2. to provide midterm feedback and assist students in developing competent performance over time.

Key Features

Several key features differentiate the fieldwork performance evaluation forms from the previous evaluations:

- The *FWPE/OTS* and the *FWPE/OTAS* are companion documents that share the same conceptual foundation, format, and rating scale. This feature helps differentiate the roles and responsibilities of the occupational therapist and occupational therapy assistant, which is helpful for sites that take both levels of students.
- The *FWPEs* can be used across and within all practice settings.

- The *FWPE*s can be adapted and customized to be used with all types and lengths of Level II fieldwork.
- Ease in use was enhanced by clarifying and reducing the number of items and providing a performance summary sheet with space for both midterm and final scores to be recorded.
- Preliminary midterm and final cutoff scores assist with evaluation of student performance over time. The evaluation forms can be used as both formative and summative evaluations.
- The rating scale was changed from a 5-point to a 4-point rating scale including descriptors of when and how often a rating would be used. The descriptors (4 = "exceeds standards," 3 = "meets standards," 2 = "needs improvement," and 1 = "unsatisfactory") reflect a measure of competency rather than global ratings (e.g., "excellent," "good").
- The *FWPE*s were designed so that students who do not meet standards on all items related to ethics and safety will not pass the fieldwork rotation.

Use of the Fieldwork Performance Evaluation Forms

Use of the *FWPE/OTS* and *FWPE/OTAS* is recommended by the AOTA COE; however, the final determination of whether to use the evaluation forms is made by the academic program in collaboration with each fieldwork site. The fieldwork performance evaluation forms were not designed, or intended to be used, to assign academic grades. It is up to the academic program professionals to determine grades. This manual assists academic fieldwork coordinators (AFWCs) and fieldwork educators in understanding

- the conceptual foundation of the evaluations,
- the research and development of the evaluations, and
- how to use the evaluations.

It is strongly recommended that all fieldwork educators and supervisors who provide input into students' performance, and the students themselves, receive education and training on these evaluations before using the *FWPE/OTS* and *FWPE/OTAS*.

CHAPTER 2

Conceptual Foundation of the Fieldwork Performance Evaluation Forms

Fieldwork is an essential component of preparing occupational therapy and occupational therapy assistant students to become entry-level occupational therapists and occupational therapy assistants. The role of fieldwork is to help students not only develop needed skills but also to become socialized into the profession and become ethical and competent occupational therapists and occupational therapy assistants who engage in daily practice that reflects the core values and beliefs of the profession (Accreditation Council for Occupational Therapy Education [ACOTE}, 1999a, 1999b; Bonello, 2001; Sabari, 1985). Regardless of the practice setting in which the student completes Level II fieldwork, entry-level competence related to the ability to engage in the occupational therapy process is the outcome of Level II fieldwork. The steps in the occupational therapy process assist occupational therapists and occupational therapy assistants to help people engage in daily occupations that they need or want to do, across all practice settings American Occupational Therapy Association [AOTA], 2002; Christiansen & Baum, 1997; Creek, 1997; Fearing & Clark, 2000; A. G. Fisher, 2001). Therefore, the conceptual foundation of the *FWPE/OTS* and the *FWPE/OTAS* was drawn from key documents of the profession that

- reflect the uniqueness of the profession (AOTA, 2002),
- clarify the purpose of fieldwork education (ACOTE, 1999a, 1999b),
- delineate the roles and responsibilities of entry-level occupational therapists and occupational therapy assistants (ACOTE, 1999a, 1999b; AOTA, 1998, 2002), and
- reflect current practice (National Board for Certification in Occupational Therapy [NBCOT], 1997).

The new fieldwork evaluation forms evaluate students' abilities to carry out the occupational therapy process in a professional and ethical manner. The forms reinforce the purpose of fieldwork, which is to develop competent entry-level generalists. Fieldwork provides students with an in-depth experience in delivering occupational therapy services to clients focusing on the application of occupation-based practice (ACOTE, 1999a, 1999b). The *Standards of Practice for Occupational Therapy* (AOTA, 1998) and ACOTE's *Standards for an Accredited Educational Program for the Occupational Therapist* (ACOTE, 1999a) and the *Standards for an Accredited Educational Program for the Occupational Therapy Assistant* (ACOTE, 1999b) all address entry-level roles and responsibilities and clearly discuss the requirements of the occupational therapist and occupational therapy assistant in implementing the occupational therapy process. Using the conceptual foundations of core educational and practice documents reviewed below allows the fieldwork performance evaluation forms to be used in all practice settings, including emerging practice areas.

Occupational Therapy Practice Framework: Domain and Process

The *Occupational Therapy Practice Framework: Domain and Process* (AOTA, 2002) provides a comprehensive overview of the domain of occupational therapy and an outline of the occupational therapy process in which occupational therapists and occupational therapy assistants engage when delivering occupational therapy services. This document replaced the *Uniform Terminology for Occupational Therapy, Third Edition* (AOTA, 1994). In the *Framework*, the primary focus of the occupational therapist and occupational therapy assistant is to assist the client (individual, group, or population) in engaging in occupations to support participation in daily life activities in a variety of contexts (AOTA, 2002). Although many health care professionals use the same problem-solving process, the "focus on occupation throughout the process makes the profession's application and use of the process unique" (AOTA, 2002, p. 613).

According to the *Framework*, the occupational therapy process includes three main components:

1. Evaluation (profile and analysis)

2. Establishing the intervention plan and the intervention plan implementation and review

3. Targeting outcomes, with the overall outcome focused on supporting engagement in occupation.

The *Framework* clearly describes how the occupational therapist, occupational therapy assistant, and client collaboratively interact throughout the entire process, keeping a major focus on *meaningful occupations*—in other words, what the client needs or wants to do. In addition to identifying the steps in the occupational therapy process, the *Framework* illustrates the clinical reasoning process that the occupational therapy practitioner uses during each step. The clinical reasoning process is the thinking behind why practitioners choose to do what they do based on evidence from the literature, the client's condition, the client's story, the practice setting, the effectiveness of past interventions, or a combination of these elements (Bridge & Twible, 1997; Mattingly, 1991; Schell, 1998).

The *Framework* emphasizes the importance of occupation-based practice and illustrates how occupation is the major focus of each step in the occupational therapy process. At the same time, the *Framework* acknowledges that the focus of occupational therapy may vary in different settings. For example, in home health care the focus is on supporting an immediate ability of the client to engage in self-care and home management occupation, whereas in a hand therapy clinic the focus may be on improving underlying client factors that will enable engagement in occupation at a later time. In addition, it is important to realize that the steps in the occupational therapy process reflect the unique context of each setting. For example, when participating in intervention planning in a school setting, the occupational therapist will collaborate with the student and other professionals in developing an individualized education program, whereas in a hospital the occupational therapist will develop a treatment plan with input from the patient. In all situations, the steps of the occupational therapy process and clinical reasoning are evident, providing a broad conceptual foundation for how occupational therapy services are delivered to clients in any setting. This broad conceptual foundation became the structure for organizing the *FWPE/OTS* and the *FWPE/OTAS*.

Roles and Responsibilities of Entry-Level Occupational Therapists and Occupational Therapy Assistants

In the occupational therapy profession there is general agreement as to the major steps in the occupational therapy process; however, there is less agreement and clarity when attempting to define entry-level practice. The intent of entry-level practice is clarified in the *Standards for an Accredited Educational Program for the Occupational Therapist* (ACOTE, 1999a), *Standards for an Accredited Educational Program for the Occupational Therapy Assistant* (ACOTE, 1999b), and the *Standards of Practice for Occupational Therapy* (AOTA, 1998). ACOTE sets the standards for education programs that include fieldwork education. The minimum standard set is to develop the basic skills needed for entry-level competence for the occupational therapist and the occupational therapy assistant. *Entry-level* is defined as being "prepared to begin generalist practice as an occupational therapy practitioner with less than 1 year of experience" (AOTA, 1999a, p. 590). *Competency* is defined as having "the requisite ability/qualities and capacity to function in a professional environment" (AOTA, 1999a, p. 590). Table 1 compares and contrasts what the entry-level occupational therapists and occupational therapy assistants must be prepared to do. After completion of an education program that includes fieldwork, entry-level occupational therapists and occupational therapy assistants should possess basic skills as direct care providers, educators, and advocates for consumers and the profession. In addition, entry-level occupational therapists should possess basic skills to enable them to function as consultants, managers of personnel and resources, and researchers.

Standards of Practice for Occupational Therapy

The AOTA *Standards of Practice for Occupational Therapy* (1998) identify the minimum requirements for occupational therapists and occupational therapy assistants for the delivery of client-centered occupational therapy services. The minimum requirements are outlined in eight standards, or areas: (a) professional standards and responsibilities, (b) referral, (c) screening, (d) evaluation, (e) intervention planning, (f) intervention, (g) transition services, and (h) discontinuation. Exhibit 1 highlights key behaviors under each area. The "professional standards and responsibilities" subset addresses ethical practice and professional behaviors, and all the other areas are aspects of the occupational therapy process used in all practice settings. Note the strong relationship between the minimum requirements of the education standards and the practice standards; both reflect the ability of occupa-

Table 1. Comparison of Requirements for Entry-Level Occupational Therapists and Occupational Therapy Assistants

Entry-level occupational therapists must be prepared to	Entry-level occupational therapy assistants must be prepared to
• Be generalists, prepared to practice in a variety of settings • Achieve entry-level competence • Articulate, apply, and justify principles, intervention approaches, and rationales related to occupation • Supervise and collaborate with occupational therapy assistants • Keep current with best practices • Uphold the ethical standards, values, and attitudes of the occupational therapy profession • Be effective consumers of research and knowledge	• Be generalists, prepared to practice in a variety of settings • Achieve entry-level competence • Articulate and apply principles, intervention approaches, and rationales related to occupation • Work under the supervision of and in cooperation with occupational therapists • Keep current with best practices • Uphold the ethical standards, values, and attitudes of the profession

Note. From the American Occupational Therapy Association (1999b, p. 575; 1999c, p. 583).

tional therapists and occupational therapy assistants to carry out the occupational therapy process in an ethical and professional manner.

NBCOT Practice Analysis

Review of the 1997 practice analysis published by NBCOT (which was the most current practice analysis at the time of the development of the *FWPE/OTS* and *FWPE/OTAS*) emphasized the same requirements and competencies identified in the ACOTE educational standards and the *Standards of Practice for Occupational Therapy.* One of NBCOT's responsibilities is the initial certification of occupational therapists and occupational therapy assistants, certifying/verifying that the individuals who pass the examination meet the entry-level competencies to practice as an occupational therapist or occupational therapy assistant. A *practice analysis* is a method used to ensure that a credentialing examination reflects current practice. The NBCOT practice analysis results identified the major functions of occupational therapy (i.e., the occupational therapy process) and the specific tasks that must be performed by occupational therapists and occupational therapy assistants to carry out these functions in practice settings. The practice analysis also identified the specific knowledge and skills one must have to competently perform these functions and tasks (see Table 2). This document became important in identifying how the occupational therapy process is implemented across practice settings by both occupational therapists and occupational therapy assistants.

In summary, throughout all of the documents reviewed, the role of occupational therapists and occu-

Exhibit 1. *Standards of Practice for Occupational Therapy:* **Key Performance Areas**

1. **Professional Standing:** Follows policies and procedures; functions according to the *AOTA Code of Ethics* and *Standards of Practice for Occupational Therapy;* identifies and pursues own professional growth and development; maintains work areas; manages one's own work schedule. (*Note:* These are some aspects of professional behaviors and aspects of service management.)

2. **Referral:** Responds to requests for services according to policies and procedures.

3. **Screening:** Screens individuals to determine the need for intervention.

4. **Evaluation:** Occupational therapist obtains and interprets data for planning and carrying out intervention; occupational therapy assistant assists with data collection.

5. **Intervention Plan:** Develops and coordinates intervention plans, including goals and methods to achieve stated goals.

6. **Intervention:** Selects, implements, and adapts intervention to meet the needs of the client; communicates and collaborates with others; documents services as required, maintaining records required by practice setting and third-party payers.

7. **Transitional Services:** Develops home and community transition programming to support performance in natural environment.

8. **Discontinuation:** Terminates services when maximum benefit is received and formulates discontinuation and follow-up plans. (*Note:* Key Performance Areas 2–8 are all aspects of the occupational therapy process that is the guiding structure of the fieldwork performance evaluations.)

Note. From American Occupational Therapy Association (1998, pp. 866–868).

Table 2. Tasks and Knowledge Identified as Requirements for Current Practice/NBCOT Practice Analysis Results

What occupational therapists and occupational therapy assistants do	What occupational therapists and occupational therapy assistants need to know
• Determine needs and priorities for interventions • Identify and design interventions • Implement interventions • Report and evaluate intervention effectiveness • Provide occupational therapy services for populations • Manage delivery of occupational therapy services • Advance effectiveness of the occupational therapy profession	• Human development and performance • Principles and strategies in the identification and evaluation of strengths and needs • Principles and strategies in intervention and treatment planning • Principles and strategies in intervention • The nature of occupation and occupational performance • Service management • His or her responsibilities as a professional

Note. From National Board for Certification in Occupational Therapy (NBCOT; 1997, pp. 7–8).

pational therapy assistants in delivering occupational therapy services is clearly delineated. Competence is the major goal of Level II fieldwork, as students learn to apply their knowledge and clinical reasoning skills while engaging in the occupational therapy process.

The new *FWPE/OTS* and the *FWPE/OTAS* assess whether students are ready for entry-level practice by measuring their ability to engage in the occupational therapy process in a professional and ethical manner.

CHAPTER 3

Development and Pilot
Validity and Reliability Studies

This chapter reviews the background of how and why the *FWPE/OTS* and the *FWPE/OTAS* were developed, including the results of three pilot validity and reliability studies. The information in this chapter will help readers understand the design of the new fieldwork evaluation forms and will help them accurately use the *FWPEs*. After a summary of the need to update the fieldwork evaluations, a brief introduction to Rasch measurement concepts is presented. The simple Rasch model was used to guide the development of the fieldwork performance evaluation forms.

Need for Updated Fieldwork Evaluation Forms

As the practice of occupational therapy continues to change and develop, there has been and will continue to be a simultaneous need to update the evaluations used to measure Level II fieldwork student performance (Cooper & Crist, 1988; Crist & Cooper, 1988; Crocker, Muthard, Slaymaker, & Samson, 1975; Culler, 1991; Halom, 1991; Rogers & Elberth, 2000). Most recently, there has been an expansion of fieldwork into emerging practice areas (Kolodner & Hischmann, 2000) and development of different fieldwork models (O'Connor & Collier, 2000) to meet the need for fieldwork placements. In light of these changes, Accreditation Council for Occuptional Therapy Education [ACOTE] criteria for acceptable fieldwork experiences includes sites where supervision of students may be shared with on-site non-occupational therapy personnel and with off-site or part-time occupational therapists (ACOTE, 1999a, 1999b). These changes have led some to feel that the *Fieldwork Evaluation for the Occupational Therapist* (*FWE/OT;* American Occupational Therapy Association [AOTA], 1987) and the *Fieldwork Evaluation Form for Occupational Therapy Assistant Students* (*FWE/OTAS;* AOTA, 1983) are not applicable to several settings.

In addition, concerns have been expressed about how to adequately use the *FWE/OT* to rate student performance (Commission on Education [COE], AOTA, 1994). Guidelines were subsequently published (Culler, 1991; Halom, 1991; Rogers & Elberth, 2000) to help support the accurate use of the fieldwork evaluations. Rogers and Elberth (2000) cautioned both students and fieldwork educators that the 5-point scale of the *FWE/OT* may be easy to equate to the more familiar letter grade system (A, B, C) used in academic settings. Not using the scale as intended can lead to grade inflation.

No studies have examined the reliability and validity of the *FWE/OTAS* after its initial development in 1983, although two studies have examined the reliability and validity of the *FWE/OT.* In 1992, the COE of AOTA mandated a review of the fieldwork evaluations by the Fieldwork Issues Committee to explore these concerns. In particular, the review, which was conducted by Stutz-Tanenbaum et al. (1993), examined the appropriateness and relevance of the items across practice areas and sites and the system of grading used in the *FWE/OT.* Using simple Rasch analysis, Stutz-Tanenbaum et al. examined 240 fieldwork evaluations from four occupational therapy education programs. The results indicated that (a) most items from all three categories of Performance, Judgment, and Attitude were too easy; (b) there was considerable overlap of concepts among categories, resulting in very high correlations among the total scores for the three categories, indicating that the items may represent a single factor rather than three separate factors; and (c) the evaluation failed to discriminate levels of student competency. In addition, the way the rating scale was used resulted in inflated student scores. Recommendations included (a) changing the rating scale from a 5-point scale to a 2-point scale; (b) reducing the number of items to eliminate overlap; (c) reconsidering the terminology with regard to compatibility with nonmedical settings; (d) devising only two scales related to the delivery of the occupational therapy process and professional behaviors instead of the three scales related to Performance, Judgment, and Attitude; and (e) identifying a way to gather specifics about the setting and supervisor to assist with adjusting student scores to reflect differences across settings (Stutz-Tanenbaum et al., 1993). The results of Stutz-Tanenbaum et al.'s study were later supported by Kirchner et al. (2001), who also reported that the scales (Performance, Judgment, and Attitude) might represent a single factor rather than three separate factors. Kirchner et al. also suggested that the number of items be reduced.

Simple Rasch Model

The simple Rasch model is a modern test theory model of measurement (Andrich, 1988; Masters & Keeves, 1999) that is being more commonly used in the field of rehabilitation to develop and validate assessments (Coster, Denney, Haltiwanger, & Haley, 1998; A. G. Fisher, 2001; A. G. Fisher et al., 1994; Haley & Ludlow, 1992; Velozo, Kielhofner, & Lai, 1999). Some of the advantages of using Rasch measurement methods to evaluate students' performance of entry-level competencies include the following:

- A key assumption of the simple Rasch model is that a single construct—in the case of the *FWPEs*, entry-level competency—can be measured along a single continuum with the range of competencies arranged in order from easier to harder. For example, implementing an intervention is an easier competency to achieve than clearly articulating the rationale for selecting the intervention (which is a harder, more complex competency, requiring greater integration of concepts). The key competencies required of entry-level occupational therapists and occupational therapy assistants, identified by the profession, became the starting point for conceptualizing a single construct of entry-level competency, recognizing that some of these competencies are easier to reach and some are harder.

- There are two basic assertions or claims that are fundamental to the simple Rasch model: (a) the easy-to-reach competency items are more likely to be reached by all students and (b) the more competent the student, the more likely the student will reach competency on easy-to-reach as well as hard-to-reach competency items. One way of investigating whether the measurement tool (the fieldwork performance evaluation form) follows the basic assertions fundamental to the simple Rasch model is to examine the curves that show the probability of receiving a certain rating. Figure 1 illustrates the 4-point scale of the *FWPE/OTAS*

that is working well to differentiate students' abilities. Students' abilities or competencies are shown along the horizontal axis and can range from –9.0 to 9.0 on a log-odds probability units (logit) scale. A *logit scale* is a scale in which students' ability raw scores are transformed into equal interval units called *logits* (Bond & Fox, 2001). The vertical axis indicates the probability of getting a particular score. Probabilities range from 0 (no chance of getting a particular score) to 1 (100% chance of getting a particular score). A student with a competency falling at –3.0 logits has a probability of about 0.9 (90% chance) to get a score of 2. When the level of competency increases to 0 logits, the student has a probability of 0.5 (50% chance) of getting either a score of 2 or 3. In contrast, the most probable rating for a more-competent student (3.0 logits) is a 3 (top of the curve), and this student would not be very likely to get a score of 1, 2, or 4 (bottom of the curve). Because the *FWPEs* were developed using the simple Rasch model, one would not expect all students to score equally well across all items. However, one would expect to see a pattern in individual students' performance following the assumptions just described.

- One of the primary advantages of using the simple Rasch model is that it transforms ordinal data (the raw scores on each *FWPE* item) into interval data (competency measures of students, expressed in linearized equal units, or logits). One characteristic of a good measurement tool is that the quantity between the units of measures are equal units of like measure. For example, on an ordinal scale, such as the rating scale on the *FWPEs* (4 = "exceeds standards," 3 = "meets standards," 2 = "needs improvement," and 1 = "unsatisfactory"), going from a score of 2 to 3 represents improvement in student performance, and going from a score of 2 to 4 represents even greater improvement in performance, but it does not necessarily represent twice as much progress. By using a Rasch computer program, the students' scores are changed to equal intervals, allowing a more accurate examination on how the evaluation is working to differentiate student performance. Use of the simple Rasch measurement model to develop the *FWPEs* addresses the growing concern in the literature that traditional statistics, including means and standard deviations, cannot be applied in a valid manner to ordinal data (Merbitz, Morris, & Grip, 1989; Wright & Linacre, 1989). When using the Rasch computer program to analyze the data, it becomes possible to examine the data in much more detail. When designing evaluation tools, it is helpful to analyze the data at the level of each individual item rating by each individual rater for each individual student. Rasch measurement methods enable one to inspect data in far greater detail than traditional measurement statistics. Traditional measurement statistics primarily evaluate the data from the perspective of the sample of persons as a whole (i.e., group means, standard deviations, standard errors). In contrast, Rasch model statistics are sample free, not dependent (Bond & Fox, 2001). This means that the estimated competency measures for the students are estimated independently of the difficulty of the items included in the *FWPEs*, and the difficulties of the items are estimated independently of the competencies of the students who are evaluated. This is in contrast to traditional measurement statistics in which the sample means and standard deviation, as well as estimates of reliability and item difficulty, are dependent on the difficulties of the items or the competencies of the students.

Figure 1. Pattern of the Well-Functioning 4-Point Scale of the *FWPE/OTAS*

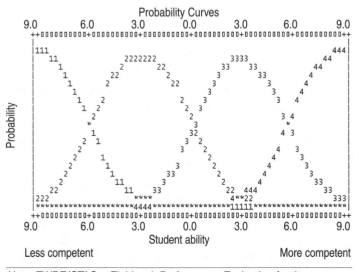

Note. FWPE/OTAS = Fieldwork Performance Evaluation for the Occupational Therapy Assistant Student.

dents. As a result, the characteristics and size of the sample become less critical when using Rasch models than when using traditional measurement statistics. In the latter case, there is a greater need for larger randomized samples that represents the target population (van de Vijver, 1986).

Development of the Forms

In addition to examining the reliability and validity of the *FWPE/OTS* and *FWPE/OTAS*, the Fieldwork Evaluation Revision Task Force reviewed literature related to competency and measurement issues (Hager & Gonczi, 1996; Neufeld & Norman, 1985; Salvatori, 1996) regarding student performance evaluations, both inside and outside the profession, including the Occupational Therapy Attribute Scale (Hubbard, 1999), the University of Alberta Occupational Therapy Student Evaluation, the Queen Margaret College Assessment of Fieldwork Studies, the Performance Evaluation of the Occupational Therapy Student (Ernest & Polatajko, 1986; Missiuna, Polatajko, & Ernest-Conibear, 1992; Polatajko, Lee, & Bossers, 1994), the Clinical Fellowship Skills Inventory (American Speech–Language–Hearing Association, 1997), and the Physical Therapist Clinical Performance Instrument (American Physical Therapy Association, 1997). This review process assisted the task force in establishing a plan for revising the fieldwork evaluations. After approval was received from the COE, the first versions of the fieldwork evaluations were designed and piloted. The characteristics incorporated into these first versions included the following:

1. The number of items was significantly reduced, and the content was broadened to reflect key competencies (rather than skills) required of entry-level occupational therapists and occupational therapy assistants in delivering occupational therapy services.

2. In addition to attempting to expand items to reflect tasks required across various fieldwork placement settings, a feature was created that allowed fieldwork educators to customize the evaluation forms to the settings by ranking the importance of each performance item. Before the start of fieldwork rotations, fieldwork educators ranked each performance item as (a) 3—"Critical": a critical element of this facility, *essential* for the achievement of entry-level competence for this

Table 3. Comparison of Scoring Methods 1 and 2

Scoring Method 1	Scoring Method 2
Overview	
Example Item: Intervention Selection	
Same rating scale used for each performance item. Each item rated on a 5-point scale.	Performance descriptions are written for each rating: Outstanding, Exceeds Standards, Meets Standards, Needs Improvement, Unsatisfactory
Selects relevant interventions directly linked to the established plan, which reflect clients' occupations (self-care, work, leisure), the factors that support and hinder performance, and the context of the service delivery setting. Develops methods and approaches through collaboration with clients, significant others, and professionals, with general supervision.	*Outstanding:* Demonstrates exceptional ability to select relevant interventions that are client-centered and occupation-based. Consistently seeks and collaborates effectively with the client, staff, and significant others.
Rating scale:	*Exceeds Standards:* Demonstrates above-average ability to select relevant interventions that are client-centered and occupation-based. Collaborates frequently with the client, staff, and significant others.
0 = Requires constant direction and assistance.	*Meets Standards:* Demonstrates average ability to select relevant interventions that are client-centered and occupation-based with general supervision. Collaborates with the client, staff, and significant others with occasional reminders.
1 = Requires considerable direction and assistance, and skill development is needed for entry-level practice. Skills need improvement.	
2 = Requires daily direction or assistance. Skill development is consistent with entry-level practice expectations.	*Needs Improvement:* Requires much prompting and guidance to select relevant interventions that are client-centered and occupation-based. Requires frequent reminders to collaborate with the client, staff, and significant others.
3 = Requires minimal direction or assistance. Skill development is just beyond entry-level practice expectations.	
4 = Requires direction or assistance similar to that of an experienced employee. Performance is outstanding, self-initiated, and highly professional.	*Unsatisfactory:* Unable to select relevant interventions that are client-centered and occupation-based. Does not collaborate with the client, staff, and significant others.

setting; (b) 2—"Important": a primary element of this facility, *significant* for the achievement of entry-level competence for this setting; or (c) 1—"Moderately Important": a supplemental element for this facility, *important* for the achievement of entry-level competence for this setting. Students' final scores were determined by multiplying the performance rating by the importance ranking.

3. Two methods of scoring were developed in an attempt to determine the format best suited for measuring entry-level performance and ease of use for fieldwork educators. The two versions (see Table 3) were based on constituency feedback and review of the literature on evaluation meth-

ods. Scoring Method 1 included various performance items that were rated on a 5-point scale. Scoring Method 2 provided behavioral descriptors of students' performance at the five levels.

Pilot Study 1

Once the *FWPE/OTAS* had been developed, reviewed by an experienced panel (including academic fieldwork coordinators [AFWCs] fieldwork educators, and recent occupational therapy assistant Level II fieldwork students) and approved by the COE, it was evaluated with a pilot study. After a convenience sample had been gathered from AFWCs of occupational therapy assistant educational programs, 225 evaluation forms using Scor-

Figure 2. Relationship Between Item Difficulty in Scoring Methods 1 and 2

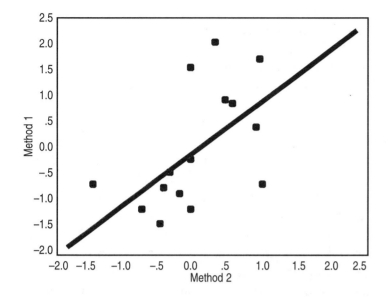

Figure 3. Relationship Between How Fieldwork Educators Rank Item Importance in Scoring Methods 1 and 2

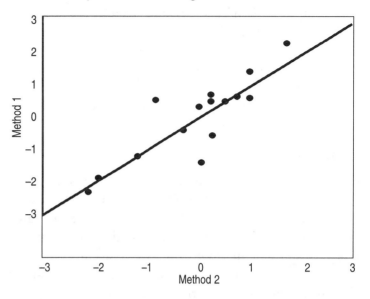

ing Method 1 and 243 evaluation forms using Scoring Method 2 were sent out with return rates of 40% and 30%, respectively. To examine whether there was a difference in the items on Scoring Methods 1 and 2 (i.e., whether the two methods were measuring the same thing), the item difficulty calibrations (statistics generated by the Rasch computer program) on Scoring Method 1 were plotted against the item difficulty calibrations on Scoring Method 2 (see Figure 2). Item difficulties that are similar between Methods 1 and 2 are located close to the diagonal control line. The farther away from the control line the items are located, the more different they are. Results indicated that the two methods of measuring student performance were not equivalent. Data from the pilot tests of the two methods, therefore, were analyzed separately.

Each item's importance ranking between the two methods of scoring was plotted to examine whether there was any agreement in what fieldwork educators perceived as important performance competencies for occupational therapy assistant students across settings (see Figure 3). Fieldwork educators ranked safety, implementation of interventions, ethics, work behaviors, and verbal communication as most important to their practice (top right-hand side of Figure 3), whereas shares what occupational therapy is, uses resources, and data gathering were perceived as least important (bottom left-hand side of Figure 3). All but two of the items (competencies) were very close to the diagonal control line, indicating that there was strong agreement across

settings. Although the use of importance weightings was intended to give items of greater importance more weight, it became apparent in retrospect that multiplying by 1, 2, or 3 is rather arbitrary and may not reflect actual differences. That is, if an item is multiplied by 2, then the data are given twice as much weight, but that item might be only slightly more important. In fact, the importance rankings only served to skew students' overall scores (importance ranking × student's rating on items = overall score). This feature was therefore eliminated in future pilot studies, because use of the simple Rasch model results in the importance of the item being reflected in the item difficulty calibration. In other words, an item's importance is reflected in the degree to which it reflects a task that is easy to achieve with competence versus a task harder to achieve with competence. These difficulties are defined by the performance of the students and not by arbitrary judgments of fieldwork educators.

Through simple Rasch analysis and qualitative feedback from fieldwork educators and students who participated in the pilot study, the following conclusions were reached:

- Neither form discriminated entry-level competency, because the rating scale was not used correctly (fieldwork educators primarily used a 3-point rating scale, never or rarely giving scores of 0 or 1).
- There were not enough items to differentiate levels of competency.
- Specificity of items was lacking.

However, both the quantitative and qualitative results indicated that Scoring Method 1 was a better and more preferred format. The COE approved repiloting the *FWPE/OTAS* after changes to the rating scale were incorporated (clarifying definitions and reducing the rating scale to a 4-point scale) and items were changed (items were added or reworded to ensure that each item measured a single task vs. multiple tasks) and the importance ranking was eliminated.

Pilot Study 2

The revised *FWPE/OTAS* was piloted a second time. Seventy-one pilot evaluation forms of 500 were returned, for a return rate of 14%. The low return rate was primarily due to the timing of the second pilot study (fewer occupational therapy assistant students were out on fieldwork). Despite the small sample size, the sample included a variety of settings that employ occupational therapy assistants and was representative of where they practice. Most of the data were reflective of where most occupational therapy assistant programs are located (the eastern United States), although there was good geographical representation from across the United States. Fieldwork educators who participated had a range of years of experience supervising students (range <1–25 years; M = 6.3 years). Analysis of the data returned using simple Rasch analysis is presented below.

Validity and reliability. Using the FACETS computer program (Linacre, 1987–2002), each student's rating on each individual item was changed into linear competency measures for students, expressed in equal interval logit units. Rasch computer programs provide statistics that include (a) item difficulty calibrations and the standard error for each calibration; (b) student competency measures and the standard error for each student's measure; (c) goodness-of-fit statistics (mean square (*MnSq*) and standardized residuals (*z*)) for each item and each student; and (d) separation indices for items and students. Mean square is a ratio of the actual score and the score expected by the simple Rasch measurement model.

The goodness-of-fit statistics provide a way to evaluate how well each item and each student demonstrated a pattern of scores expected by the simple Rasch model. For example, students who have higher competency measures but fail to get a high score on an easy item (a task that is easy for most students to perform competently) have a higher-than-expected mean square and *z* goodness-of-fit statistics.

The separation indices provide a way to evaluate how students' responses provide evidence that the items on the *FWPE*s are spread along the continuum of competency to create a scale of items with differing levels of difficulty and how well the items in the *FWPE*s divide (separate) the students into different levels of competency. The item difficulty calibrations and student competency measures have been, as mentioned earlier, linearized, by means of logistic transformation procedures, into equal interval numbers expressed in logits (Bond & Fox, 2001). When reporting the results of a simple Rasch analysis, validity and reliability are reported for both the items' and students' measures. Validity and reliability of items are described in terms of item difficulty calibrations, standard errors, goodness-of-fit statistics, and the item separation index. Similarly, validity and reliability of students' measures are described in terms of student competency measures, standard errors, goodness-of-fit statistics, and the student separation index.

Item validity and reliability. Table 4 lists the item difficulty calibrations and the goodness-of-fit statistics for the items on the *FWPE/OTAS*. The item difficulty calibrations ranged from 1.76 to –1.26 logits, which indicates a good range of items across the construct of competency. The standard errors given in column 2 of Table 4 represent the extent to which the difficulty estimate may be expected to vary, a concept that is similar to standard error in traditional test statistics. However, in traditional statistics, the standard error is only for people (not items) and is a single value estimated for the entire sample. The standard error is reported for each item calibration and each person by the Rasch analysis program. The average standard error for the scale items was 0.25 (0.40 is acceptable), which indicates good reliability of the item calibration estimates.

Closer review of the mean square fit statistics (see Table 4, columns 3–6) indicated that 21 of 23 items demonstrated acceptable goodness-of-fit or, in other words, the items fit the Rasch model assumptions. Items were judged not to demonstrate acceptable goodness-of-fit if they had mean square values ≥1.4 and an associated *z* ≥2 (Wright & Linacre, 1994). Work behaviors (*MnSq* = 1.4, *z* = 2) and self-responsibility (*MnSq* 1.5, *z* = 3) were the two items that failed to demonstrate acceptable goodness-of-fit. A detailed analysis of indi-

Table 4. *FWPE/OTAS* Item Measurements From Easier-to-Reach Competencies to Harder-to-Reach Competencies and Goodness-of-Fit Statistics

Item	Item Difficulty	SE	Infit MnSq	Infit z	Outfit MnSq	Outfit z
Cultural competence	1.76	0.27	1.3	1	1.5	1
Ethics	1.70	0.24	1.0	0	1.0	0
Responds to feedback	1.53	0.24	1.0	0	1.0	0
Interpersonal skills	1.50	0.27	1.2	1	1.2	0
Safety	1.36	0.24	1.1	0	1.2	0
Work behaviors	0.83	0.27	**1.4**	**2**	1.5	1
Therapeutic use of self	0.62	0.23	1.0	0	0.9	0
Written communication	0.44	0.23	1.0	0	1.4	1
Verbal/nonverbal communication	0.12	0.24	1.1	0	1.0	0
Self-responsibility	0.04	0.28	**1.5**	**3**	**1.5**	**2**
Implements intervention	−0.06	0.25	0.8	−1	0.7	−1
Occupational therapy/occupational therapy assistant roles	−0.25	0.26	1.2	1	1.2	0
Data gathering	−0.28	0.23	1.0	0	1.2	0
Selects intervention	−0.62	0.25	0.8	−1	0.8	−1
Activity analysis	−0.62	0.24	0.9	0	0.9	0
Evidence-based practice	−0.71	0.24	0.9	0	0.8	0
Plans intervention	−0.76	0.27	0.7	−2	0.7	−2
Reports	−0.86	0.28	0.7	−2	0.6	−2
Occupational therapy philosophy	−1.04	0.25	0.8	−1	0.7	−1
Administers assessments	−1.05	0.24	1.0	0	0.8	0
Establishes goals	−1.10	0.24	0.9	0	0.9	0
Modifies intervention plan	−1.26	0.26	0.8	−1	0.8	−1
Interprets	−1.30	0.31	0.6	−3	0.5	−3

Note. Numbers in boldface type are the items that failed to demonstrate acceptable goodness-of-fit. *FWPE/OTAS = Fieldwork Performance Evaluation for the Occupational Therapy Assistant Student.*

vidual item responses found that there was no underlying pattern of the item response misfit across different settings, indicating that the scale is equally valid across diverse settings. The separation index is a measure of reliability. In this case, the item separation of 3.79 (2.0 is acceptable; W. P. Fisher, 1993) indicated that the students did reliably separate the items into at least four levels of difficulty along the continuum of competency, from more difficult to less difficult.

Examination of the ordering of the items by difficulty, from competencies that are easier to reach to those that are harder to reach (see Table 4), revealed a logical sequence as determined by the task force and fieldwork educators who participated in reviewing the task force's work, attended preliminary workshops during the development process, or did both. Competencies that were easier to reach (positive logit values located at the top of the items in Table 4) were related to fundamentals (ethics and safety) and professional behaviors (i.e., "responds to feedback" and "interpersonal skills"), and competencies that were harder to reach (negative logit values located at the bottom of the items in Table 4) were related to sharing what occupational therapy is, administering assessments, establishing goals, and modifying intervention plans.

Student response: Validity and reliability. The student competency measures for the students ranged from 10.46 to −3.11 logits, with positive measures being associated with more competency and negative measures being associated with lower competency. As noted earlier, student goodness-of-fit statistics determine the extent to which the pattern of each student's responses

Figure 4. Comparison of Expected and Unexpected Patterns of Student Response by Goodness-of-Fit Statistics

Expected response	4	4	4	4	3	4	3	3	3	2	2	2
Unexpected response 1	4	4	3	4	3	3	3	2	3	**4**	2	**4**
Unexpected response 2	4	**2**	4	4	3	3	2	3	3	2	2	2

Competency items

Easier to reach   Harder to reach

Note. Numbers in bold type are the responses that misfit.

(scores) fit the expected pattern according to the simple Rasch model. In Figure 4, the items are ordered from left to right, from easier-to-reach competencies to harder-to-reach competencies. Recall that all students are more likely to have higher scores on easy items and lower scores on harder items. The overall expected pattern of student ability measures is illustrated in Row 1 in Figure 4. This student had higher scores on easier items and lower scores on harder items and demonstrated good fit. The student whose scores are in Row 2 unexpectedly got a high score (4) on two of the hardest items. Likewise, the student whose scores are in Row 3 unexpectedly got a lower score on an easier item. Both of these students did something unexpected by the simple Rasch model; both had higher goodness-of-fit statistics. Figure 5 indicates the difference in student response patterns between more-competent students and a less-competent student.

The number of students who failed to demonstrate acceptable goodness-of-fit was 10/113 (9%). Again, a detailed analysis on a score-by-score basis was conduct-

Figure 5. Comparison of Student Response Patterns Between More-Competent and Less-Competent Students

More-competent students	4	4	4	4	3	4	4	3	2	3	3	3	3	3
	4	4	3	3	3	3	3	2	2	3	3	2	2	2
	3	4	4	3	3	3	3	3	3	2	3	2	2	2
	3	3	3	3	2	3	2	3	2	2	2	2	2	2
Less-competent students	3	3	2	2	2	2	2	1	2	2	1	2	1	1

Competency items

Easier to reach   Harder to reach

ed to see whether there was any underlying pattern among the misfitting students—in other words, to identify the disruption or the source of the error in the expected pattern. In the case of the *FWPE/OTAS,* no pattern was found across settings, raters, or items. The average standard error was 0.69 (0.40 is acceptable). To reduce the standard error, one would need to reduce the amount of off targeting, which is discussed below, and possibly increase the number of items. Despite a high average standard error, the *student separation index* (the statistic that indicates how well the items spread out the students to differentiate levels of competency) of 3.22 (2.0 is acceptable) indicated that the scale does reliably separate the students into at least four levels of competency.

In addition to the validity and reliability of the items and students separately, the relationship between the item difficulties and student measures was examined. Even though the separation indices for the items and students were acceptable, a review of the placement of item difficulties relative to student competency measures revealed a concept called *off targeting.* Figure 6 gives a visual picture of the difficulty of the items (easier-to-reach competencies to harder-to-reach competencies) relative to the students' competency measures. The student competency measures (on the left-hand side of the figure), viewed from top to bottom, illustrate the range of students' performance from the more-competent students to the less-competent students. On the right-hand side of the figure is the range of items from easier-to-reach competencies (at the top) to harder-to-reach competencies (at the bottom). Notice how the majority of the students are located above most of the items. This pattern of off targeting is observed when fieldwork educators do not follow the scoring criteria and therefore score students' performance too leniently. Closer examination of the percentage of use of each of the ratings in the scale supports this pattern (4 = "exceeds standards," 29%; 3 = "meets standards," 58%; 2 = "needs improvement," 13%; and 1 = "unsatisfactory," 0%). Percentages of use are based on midterm and final scores.

Finally, and further supportive of a tendency for fieldwork educators to be too lenient, a review of qualitative data from fieldwork educators who participated in the pilot study indicated that they were not comfortable with students not passing at midterm. If the *FWPE/OTAS* is to be used properly, then fieldwork

Figure 6. Relative Positioning of Student Scores to Item Difficulty on the FWPE/OTAS

	Student Competency Measures	Item Difficulty Calibrations
Logits	More Competent	Easier-to-Reach Competencies
10	***	
	*	
9	*	
	*	
8	**	
	**	
	****	
7	*	
	***	
	*****	
6	*******	
	***	
	*********	
5	**	
	****	
	*****	
4	*****	
	********	
	******	
3	*********	
	**	
	**	
2	*	
	****	###
	***	##
1	***	#
	*****	#
		#
0	*****	###
		##
		####
−1	*	####
	**	##
−2		
	*	
−3	*	
−4	Less Competent	Harder-to-Reach Competencies

Note. * = 1, # = 1. FWPE/OTAS = Fieldwork Performance Evaluation for the Occupational Therapy Assistant Student.

educators need to be comfortable with (a) giving students lower scores at midterm and (b) knowing that a student may have an "unsatisfactory performance" at midterm but have high enough scores to pass at the final evaluation period. More important, fieldwork educators need to be comfortable with the idea that students, in general, do not have unusually high competencies, ones that (as scored) appear to exceed that of an experienced occupational therapy assistant.

To promote proper use of the evaluation form and rating scale,

- cutoff scores were developed to help fieldwork educators better judge students' competency levels relative to the minimum expected levels of competency at midterm and at final, and
- training is recommended to ensure that fieldwork educators and students understand and conceptualize that student performance or competency develops over time.

The preliminary midterm and final cutoff scores were determined by examining where students who did not meet expectations were scoring as well as the pattern of scoring across all students both at midterm and final. The hope is that as long as the student is performing satisfactorily and is meeting at least the minimum requirements, the fieldwork educators will no longer be tempted to further inflate student ratings. Addressing these two issues should help reduce the high standard errors and off targeting reported above.

The correlation between Rasch ability measures and the fieldwork educators' perceptions of students' readi-

Table 5. Occupational Therapy Assistant Fieldwork Educators' Perceptions of the FWPE/OTAS

Qualitative questions related to design and use of the FWPE/OTAS	% Agree	% Disagree
Purpose/scoring clear	77	4
Format clear	83	3
Sequence logical	83	1
Scale simple	81	3
Scale differentiates	73	11
Reflects current/future practice	76	9
Measures entry-level competencies	83	3
Can use across settings	79	6

Note. FWPE/OTAS = Fieldwork Performance Evaluation for the Occupational Therapy Assistant Student.

ness for entry-level practice (i.e., exceeds entry-level, meets entry-level, or is below entry-level) was $r = .70$, which indicated a clear correlation between the fieldwork educators' perceptions and how students scored on the *FWPE/OTAS*. Descriptive data revealed that 39% of the students who participated in the pilot study preferred the pilot version of the *FWPE/OTAS*, whereas 27% preferred the *FWE/OTAS*. Thirty-four percent did not respond. Fieldwork educators clearly reported a stronger preference for the pilot version of the *FWPE/OTAS* (61% preferred the new *FWPE*, 16% preferred the *FWE/OTAS*, and 23% did not respond). Fieldwork educators' responses to specific questions related to the design and use of the *FWPE/OTAS* are reported in Table 5.

Pilot Study 3

After Pilot Study 1 with the *FWPE/OTAS* was completed and mistakes had been learned from, the *FWPE/OTS* items and scale were developed. The *FWPE/OTS* version to be piloted was reviewed by an experienced panel (including AFWCs, fieldwork educators, and recent occupational therapy Level II fieldwork students) and was approved by the COE. Piloting of the *FWPE/OTS* was recruited at the same time as the second pilot test of the *FWPE/OTAS*. A convenience sample was obtained through advertising on the AOTA Clinical and Academic Fieldwork Educators' listserve and contacting AFWCs of occupational therapy educational programs. Three hundred thirty-two *FWPE/OTS* evaluations (out of 1,340) were returned, for a return rate of 25%. The evaluation forms returned came from a variety of settings that were representative of where occupational therapists practice and where fieldwork is completed (36% hospital, 20.6% schools, 16.3% mixed [more than one setting], 5.2% community, 3.4% nursing home, 2.8% private practice, 0.6% residential, 6.5% other). There was good geographical representation from across the United States, with a larger portion coming from the east, where more occupational therapy educational programs are located. Fieldwork educators who participated were an experienced group of occupational therapists (years practicing ranged from 1–43, $M = 11.7$) and had a range of years of experience supervising students (range: <1–34; $M = 7.32$). A majority of the students who participated were on their second fieldwork placement at the time of the pilot study (8% were on their first placement, 43% were on their second

placement, 9% were on their third placement, and 3.4% were on their fourth placement). An analysis of the data returned based on simple Rasch analysis is presented below.

Item validity and reliability. Table 6 lists the item difficulty calibrations and goodness-of-fit statistics for the items on the *FWPE/OTS*. The item difficulty calibrations (the estimate of how difficult the item was for the students) ranged from 2.18 to –1.52 logits (see column 1, Table 6), which indicates a good range of items across the construct of competency. The standard errors given in column 2 of Table 6 represent the extent to which the difficulty estimate may be expected to vary, a concept that is similar to standard error in traditional test statistics. In traditional statistics, the standard error is only for people (not the items) and is a single value estimated for the entire sample. The average standard error for the scale items was 0.11 (0.4 is acceptable), which indicates good reliability of the item calibration estimates.

Closer review of the mean square fit statistics (see Table 6, columns 3–6) indicated that 41 of 42 items demonstrated acceptable goodness-of-fit. Items were judged not to demonstrate acceptable goodness-of-fit if they had a $MnSq \geq 1.4$ and an associated $z \geq 2$ (Wright & Linacre, 1994). Legible written communication ($MnSq = 1.5$ and $z = 7$) was the item that failed to demonstrate acceptable goodness-of-fit. A detailed analysis of individual item responses found that there was no underlying pattern of the item response misfit across different settings or time of score (midterm or final), indicating that the scale is equally valid across diverse settings and at both midterm and final.

As stated earlier, the separation index is another measure of reliability. In the case of the *FWPE/OTS*, the item separation of 8.98 (2.0 is acceptable; W. P. Fisher, 1993) indicated that students do reliably separate the items into at least nine levels of difficulty along the continuum of competency, from more to less.

Examination of the ordering of the items by difficulty, from easier-to-reach competencies to harder-to-reach competencies (see Table 6), revealed a logical sequence as determined by the task force and fieldwork educators who participated in reviewing the task force's work, attended preliminary workshops during the development process, or did both. Easier-to-reach competencies (positive logit values located at the top of the items in Table 6) were related to fundamentals (ethics and safety) and professional behaviors (i.e., "responds

Table 6. *FWPE/OTS* Item Measurements From Easier-to-Reach Competencies to Harder-to-Reach Competencies and Goodness-of-Fit Statistics

Item	Item Difficulty	SE	Infit MnSq	z	Outfit MnSq	z
Positive interpersonal skills	2.18	0.12	1.2	2	1.3	1
Responds to feedback	2.03	0.12	1.1	1	1.0	0
Respects diversity	1.89	0.11	1.1	0	1.0	0
Adheres to ethics	1.67	0.11	1.0	0	1.1	0
Collaborates with supervisor	1.42	0.12	1.2	2	1.2	1
Consistent work behavior	1.28	0.11	1.2	2	1.2	1
Safety—uses judgment	1.28	0.12	1.2	2	1.5	3
Safety—adheres to safety regulations	1.23	0.11	1.0	0	1.5	3
Takes responsibility for self	1.20	0.12	1.3	4	1.3	1
Time management	0.86	0.12	1.3	4	1.5	3
Legible written communication	0.85	0.13	**1.5**	**7**	**1.8**	**5**
Implements client-centered intervention	0.67	0.11	0.8	−3	0.7	−2
Implements occupation-based intervention	0.44	0.11	0.8	−2	0.8	−2
Selects relevant occupations	0.17	0.11	0.9	−1	0.8	−2
Produces work in expected time frame	0.14	0.11	1.2	2	1.1	1
Clear documentation	0.00	0.10	0.9	0	0.9	−1
Accomplishes organizational goals	−0.12	0.10	1.0	0	1.0	0
Communicates using verbal–nonverbal methods	−0.13	0.11	1.1	2	1.1	1
Documents intervention	−0.14	0.11	0.9	−2	0.8	−2
Collaborates with client	−0.20	0.10	1.1	1	1.2	1
Uses language appropriate to recipient	−0.28	0.11	0.9	−1	0.9	−1
Documents results of evaluation	−0.30	0.10	1.0	0	0.9	−1
Articulates occupational therapy values and beliefs	−0.38	0.10	1.0	0	1.0	0
Obtains necessary information	−0.39	0.10	1.0	0	1.0	0
Communicates role of occupational therapist	−0.44	0.10	1.0	0	0.9	0
Articulates rationale for intervention	−0.51	0.12	0.7	−4	0.7	−4
Administers assessments	−0.55	0.11	1.1	1	1.1	1
Articulates rationale for evaluation	−0.55	0.11	0.8	−3	0.7	−4
Articulates value of occupation	−0.59	0.10	0.9	−1	0.9	−1
Modifies approach and occupation	−0.59	0.10	1.0	0	0.9	0
Selects occupations that motivate	−0.60	0.10	1.0	0	1.0	0
Understands cost and funding	−0.77	0.10	1.1	1	1.1	0
Collaborates with the occupational therapy assistant	−0.83	0.11	1.1	1	1.1	0
Determines occupational profile	−0.90	0.12	0.7	−4	0.7	−4
Adjusts assessment procedure	−0.91	0.11	0.9	−2	0.8	−2
Establishes plan	−1.01	0.11	0.8	−2	0.8	−2
Assesses client/contextual factors	−1.02	0.11	0.7	−4	0.7	−4
Updates/terminates intervention plan	−1.05	0.11	0.9	−2	0.8	−2
Utilizes evidence to support intervention	−1.08	0.10	0.9	−1	0.9	0
Interprets evaluation results	−1.12	0.11	0.8	−3	0.8	−3
Selects relevant assessment methods	−1.34	0.11	0.9	−2	0.9	−1
Assigns responsibility to the occupational therapy assistant	−1.52	0.11	1.0	0	1.0	0

Note. FWPE/OTS = Fieldwork Performance Evaluation for the Occupational Therapy Student. Numbers in bold type are the items that failed to demonstrate acceptable goodness-of-fit.

to feedback" and "interpersonal skills"), and the harder-to-reach competencies (negative logit values located at the bottom of the items in Table 6) were related to the more difficult tasks of evaluating (selecting assessments and interpreting results) and intervening (updating or terminating intervention) and managing (assigning responsibilities to the occupational therapy assistant).

Student response: Validity and reliability. The student competency measures ranged from 10.49 to −4.16 logits, with positive measures being associated with more competency and negative measures associated with lower competency. As noted earlier, student goodness-of-fit statistics determine the extent to which the pattern of students' responses (scores) fit the expected pattern according to the simple Rasch model. The number of students who failed to demonstrate acceptable goodness-of-fit was 10% (1,445/13,944). Again, detailed analysis completed on a score-by-score basis was done to see if there was any underlying pattern among misfitting students, an identifiable disruption or source of error in the expected pattern. In the case of the *FWPE/OTS,* no pattern was found across settings, raters, or items.

The average standard error was 0.49 (0.40 is acceptable), which is slightly high. Again, to reduce the standard error one would need to reduce the amount of off targeting, which is discussed below. Despite the slightly high average standard error, the student separation index of 4.55 (2.0 is acceptable) indicated that the items do reliably separate the students into at least five levels of competency. As described earlier regarding the *FWPE/OTAS,* despite the acceptable separation indices for the items and students, a review of the placement of item difficulties relative to student competency measures again reveals off targeting. Figure 7 gives a visual picture of the relative difficulty of the items (easier-to-reach competencies vs. harder-to-reach competencies) relative to students' competency measures for the *FWPE/OTS.* The student competency measures (on the left side of the figure), viewed from top to bottom, illustrate the range of students' performance, from the more-competent students to the less-competent students. On the right side of the figure is the range of items, from easier-to-reach competencies (at the top) to harder-to-reach competencies (at the bottom). Notice how the majority of the students are located above most of the items. Remember that the pattern of off targeting can be caused when the fieldwork educator does not follow the scoring criteria

Figure 7. Relative Positioning of Student Scores to Item Difficulty on the *FWPE/OTS*

Logits	Student Competency Measures — More Competent	Item Difficulty Calibrations — Easier-to-Reach Competencies
10	** .	
9	* .	
	* .	
8	* .	
	* .	
	***	
7	**** .	
	** .	
	***** .	
6	**** .	
	*****	
	******	
5	*** .	
	*** .	
	*******	
4	***** .	
	******* .	
	***** .	
3	*****	#
	**** .	# #
	******** .	#
2	**	# # # #
	** .	# #
	**** .	#
1	***	# #
	**** .	# # # #
	**	# # # # #
0	* .	# # # # # # #
	* .	# # # # # #
	* .	#
−1	.	#
−2	.	
−3	.	
−4	.	
−5	Less Competent	Harder-to-Reach Competencies

Note. * = 5   . = 1   # = 1. FWPE/OTS = Fieldwork Performance Evaluation for the Occupational Therapy Student.

and therefore scores students' performance too leniently. Closer examination of the percentage of use of each of the ratings in the scale again supports this pattern (4 = "exceeds standards," 34%; 3 = "meets standards," 56%; 2 = "needs improvement," 10%; and 1 = "unsatisfactory," 0%). Percentages of use are based on midterm and final scores.

Finally, further supporting a tendency for fieldwork educators to be too lenient, review of qualitative data from fieldwork educators who participated in the pilot study again indicated that they were not comfortable with students not passing at midterm. If the *FWPE/OTS* is to be used properly, fieldwork educators need to be comfortable with (a) giving students lower scores at midterm and (b) knowing that a student may have an "unsatisfactory performance" at midterm but have high enough scores to pass at the end of the fieldwork rotation. More important is that fieldwork educators need to be comfortable with the idea that students, in general, do not have unusually high competencies, ones that (as scored) appear to exceed that of an experienced occupational therapist.

To promote proper use of the evaluation form and rating scale,

- cutoff scores were developed to help fieldwork educators better judge students' competency levels relative to the minimum expected levels of competency at midterm and at final, and
- training is recommended to ensure that fieldwork educators and students understand and conceptu-

Figure 8. Rasch Ability Measures by Order of Fieldwork (FW) Placement

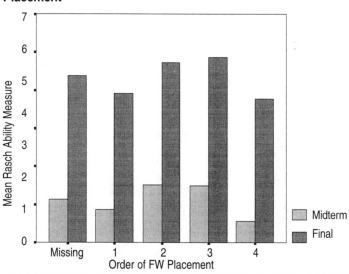

Table 7. Occupational Therapy Fieldwork Educators' Perceptions of the *FWPE/OTS*

Qualitative questions related to design and use of the *FWPE/OTS*	% Agree	% Disagree
Purpose/scoring clear	77	9
Format clear	80	7
Sequence logical	83	4
Scale simple	72	15
Scale differentiates	60	26
Reflects current/future practice	76	10
Measures entry-level competencies	75	10
Can use across settings	70	15

Note. FWPE/OTS = Fieldwork Performance Evaluation for the Occupational Therapy Student.

alize that student performance or competency develops over time.

The preliminary midterm and final cutoff scores were determined by examining where students who did not meet expectations were scoring as well as the pattern of scoring across all students both at midterm and final. The hope is that, as long as students are performing satisfactorily and are meeting at least the minimum requirements, the fieldwork educators will no longer be tempted to further inflate students' ratings. Addressing these two issues should help reduce the high standard errors and off targeting reported earlier.

Further examination of Rasch ability measures by order of fieldwork placement (first, second, third, and fourth) showed that students' performance ability measures clearly improved from midterm to the final across all fieldwork placements, thus indicating that the evaluation measures performance over time (see Figure 8). The correlation between Rasch ability measures and fieldwork educators' perceptions of students' readiness for entry-level practice (exceeds entry-level, meets entry-level, or is below entry-level) was $r = .6$, which indicated a clear correlation between the fieldwork educators' perceptions and how the students scored on the *FWPE/OTS*. Descriptive data revealed that 41% of the students who participated in the pilot study preferred the pilot version of the *FWPE/OTS*, whereas 29% preferred the *FWE/OT*. Thirty percent did not respond. Fieldwork educators' responses to specific questions related to the design and use of the *FWPE/OTS* are reported in Table 7.

On the basis of the results of the second and third pilot studies, final changes to the wording of items and rating scale were incorporated, resulting in the final versions of the *FWPE/OTAS* and *FWPE/OTS* that were adopted by the COE in August 2002. Modification in wording ensured consistency between the companion documents when possible and congruency with the language in the *Occupational Therapy Practice Framework* (AOTA, 2002).

Preliminary examination of both the *FWPE/OTAS* and the *FWPE/OTS* indicate that the evaluations are well-functioning tools that measure entry-level competency of occupational therapy students and occupational therapy assistant students across practice settings. In addition, fieldwork educators felt that the evaluation forms are user friendly and reflect current practice. The task force recommends continued examination of the reliability and validity of the *FWPEs*, particularly as practice continues to evolve.

CHAPTER 4

Using the Fieldwork Performance Evaluation Forms

The *FWPE/OTS* and the *FWPE/OTAS* are companion documents that share the same format, rating scale, and scoring procedure. This chapter includes a brief description of the evaluation format, a description of the content of the *FWPE/OTS* and *FWPE/OTAS* items (including suggestions for site-specific objectives), and an explanation of the procedure for scoring student performance. Readers are encouraged to refer to the evaluation forms found in Appendixes A and B while reviewing this chapter.

Format of the *FWPEs*

Cover sheet. The front page of the *FWPEs* includes space for identifying information and is where students' final scores and summary comments are noted. Space is provided for signatures of two raters, to allow for types of fieldwork structures in which there may be more than one supervisor/educator (i.e., in a setting where the occupational therapy fieldwork educator is not on site or where there is shared supervision).

Overview/instructions. Following a summary of the purpose and design of the *FWPEs*, the use of the evaluation forms and directions for rating students' performance are clearly identified. It is important to note that site-specific objectives need to be developed to accurately and effectively assess students' competence.

Organization of items. The items on the *FWPEs* are organized into sections that delineate the major competencies required to carry out the occupational therapy process in a professional and ethical manner. The data in Table 8 delineate the number of items under each section included on the *FWPE/OTS* and the *FWPE/OTAS* and clearly highlights the similarities of the companion documents.

Space for fieldwork educators' comments. Students benefit from supervisors' written comments, as feedback enhances students' professional development. Space for comments at midterm and at the conclusion of the fieldwork rotation is found at the end of each major section. Fieldwork educators use this space to provide feedback to (a) clarify ratings given and (b) identify students' areas of strength and areas that need improvement.

Performance rating summary sheet. At the end of the *FWPEs* are the Performance Rating Summary Sheets. Ratings on each item at midterm and the final are transferred onto the summary sheet to provide a clear picture of the students' progress toward entry-level proficiency over time.

Glossary. A glossary that defines key terms is included with the *FWPEs*. The language of the evaluation forms reflects terms from current education and practice documents (Accreditation Council for Occupational Therapy Education [ACOTE], 1999a, 1999b; American Occupational Therapy Association [AOTA], 1998, 2002; see also chapter 2). Use of the glossary ensures that all fieldwork educators are using the same definitions when evaluating students' performance and helps both students and fieldwork educators understand the scope of the competency areas being assessed.

Becoming familiar with the terms used on the *FWPEs* and comparing the terms to the everyday language used at the site assists fieldwork educators in using the evaluation forms. For example, the term *occupation* is being used more consistently in the profession

Table 8. Overview of Fieldwork Performance Evaluation Items

Section	No. Items FWPE/OTS	No. Items FWPE/OTAS
Fundamentals of practice	3	3
Basic tenets	4	3
Evaluation/screening	10	5
Intervention	9	6
Management of occupational therapy services	5	0
Communication	4	2
Professional behaviors	7	6

Note. FWPE/OTS = Fieldwork Performance Evaluation for the Occupational Therapy Student; FWPE/OTAS = Fieldwork Performance Evaluation for the Occupational Therapy Assistant Student.

and is found throughout the evaluation forms. In the glossary, *occupation* is defined as

> groups of activities and tasks of everyday life, named, organized and given value and meaning by individuals and a culture; occupation is everything people do to occupy themselves, including looking after themselves (self-care), enjoying life (leisure), and contributing to the social and economic fabric of their communities (productivity); the domain of concern and the therapeutic medium of occupational therapy. (Townsend, 1997, p. 181)

The concepts addressed in the definition of occupation, however, may be described using different terms. For example, the term *purposeful activity* may be used to describe the medium used in the facility, or the term *activities of daily living* (ADL; encompassing self-care, work, and leisure) may be used instead of *occupation* to address the outcome of therapy.

Item Content

The items on the *FWPEs* address the essential competencies required of entry-level occupational therapists and occupational therapy assistants to practice safe and effective occupational therapy as well as the reasoning that guides their actions. Each section of the *FWPEs* is described below, highlighting the intent of the items and giving examples of how one can measure the competency being assessed by clarifying expectations through written objectives. Developing site-specific objectives allows fieldwork educators to (a) identify the specific competencies that students must demonstrate to pass the fieldwork rotation and (b) clarify how students will demonstrate competencies for objectives that may not be a part of the daily activities in the setting. In addition to the examples given below, chapter 5 gives additional objectives for four case scenarios illustrating how the *FWPEs* can be individualized and used across various practice settings and sites.

When reviewing each item, keep in mind that the difficulty of the items varies from basic to complex. For example, "implementing intervention" is a basic competency that students generally achieve before being able to clearly articulate the rationale for selecting the intervention (a more complex competency). For a more in-depth explanation, refer to the discussion of the ordering of items from easier-to-reach competencies to harder-to-reach competencies for both the *FWPE/OTS* and *FWPE/OTAS* items in chapter 3.

Fundamentals of practice. The Fundamentals of Practice section includes three items related to ethical and safe practice and is generally the same on both the *FWPE/OTS* and *FWPE/OTAS*. At the final, every student must pass all items in this section to successfully complete the fieldwork experience. Ethical and safe practice is a mandatory entry-level competency for all occupational therapy practitioners. Thus, if students do not pass the three items, then they do not pass the fieldwork rotation.

Ethical practice includes adhering to the AOTA *Occupational Therapy Code of Ethics (2000)* and site-specific policies and procedures. Examples of ethical practice include such behaviors as not talking about patients in the hospital cafeteria at any time, and not taking official documentation outside of the facility. These behaviors are clear examples of how a site can state the expectations for performance through writing site-specific objectives; then both fieldwork educators and students fully understand the expectations for successfully passing the fieldwork rotation. Ethics for occupational therapy students also include issues related to human subject research, when relevant.

Safe practice involves adhering to safety regulations and applying sound judgment when implementing the occupational therapy process. Four examples of site-specific objectives include the following:

1. Uses transfer belts during all transfers.
2. Keeps sharps objects secure at all times.
3. Consistently monitors residents during community outings.
4. Sets limits to prevent undesirable client behavior.

Example Objectives 1 and 2 are written for an acute medical setting; Example 1 is applicable in a physical disability setting, and Example 2 is applicable in an acute mental health setting. Example 3 could be applicable for several settings, such as a state psychiatric hospital, a community mental health center, or a community reintegration program for clients with head injuries. Example 4 could apply to any setting, including a school system if the term *client* were changed to *student*.

Basic tenets. The items found in the Basic Tenets section address the philosophical concepts of the profession and the roles of the occupational therapist and occupational therapy assistant. Items in this section are similar on both the *FWPE/OTS* and *FWPE/OTAS* and require students to be able to share with others

- what occupational therapy is,

- what occupational therapists and occupational therapy assistants do, and
- what the values and beliefs of the profession are (i.e., how and why occupation is used as a means and an end; how and why occupational therapy practitioners are client-centered).

Table 9 compares the Basic Tenets items on the *FWPE/OTS* and the *FWPE/OTAS*. Note that for occupational therapy assistant students, the ability to incorporate evidence-based practice concepts is assessed under one item found in the Basic Tenets section. In contrast, occupational therapy students are assessed on the ability to incorporate evidence-based practice concepts with several items in the Evaluation/Screening and Intervention sections (see items 9, 16, 17, 19, and 26); therefore, a single item related to evidence-based practice is not listed. This reflects the difference in knowledge and performance expectations for occupational therapy students and occupational therapy assistant students.

In a setting where both levels of practitioners are not employed, site-specific objectives need to be written to clearly describe how students will demonstrate their ability to communicate the role of occupational therapist and occupational therapy assistant. The item is included because an entry-level practice requirement for occupational therapy students and occupational therapy assistant students are to be prepared to work in cooperation with each other (ACOTE, 1999a, 1999b). Knowing the roles of both levels of practitioners is a beginning step toward reaching this entry-level requirement. Fieldwork is a natural learning environment in which students begin to gather this knowledge. Discussion in each fieldwork setting will help students generalize knowl-

edge and be prepared for practice. Some examples of objectives include the following:

- The student presents an in-service presentation to rehabilitation staff on the potential role of the occupational therapy assistant in a like setting.
- During the midterm evaluation meeting, the student describes to the fieldwork educator the role of the occupational therapy assistant.
- The student reports on the role of the occupational therapy assistant from a site visit he or she has completed.

The student's abilities to share the philosophical values and beliefs of the profession can be assessed if objectives are developed that clarify when and how students will share this information. Examples of site-specific objectives for items in this section include the following:

- When defining *occupational therapy*, explains the uniqueness of occupational therapy services in terms understandable to clients and families.
- Presents results of occupational therapy services during meetings using language that clearly reflects the domain of occupational therapy.
- Provides an in-service presentation to ancillary staff about the role of occupational therapy.

Evaluation/screening. The items in the Evaluation/Screening section address competencies such as gathering, interpreting, planning, and reporting information related to the domain of occupational therapy practice. Table 10 provides a comparison of the Evaluation/Screening items on the *FWPE/OTS* and *FWPE/OTAS*. Occupational therapy assistant students establish service competency and work in collaboration with occupational therapists when performing screening and evalu-

Table 9. Comparison of Basic Tenets Items in the *FWPE/OTS* and *FWPE/OTAS*

Item	FWPE/OTS	FWPE/OTAS
Articulates the values and beliefs of the occupational therapy profession.	X	X
Articulates the value of occupation as a method and desired outcome.	X	Incorporated into Values and Beliefs section
Communicates the role of the occupational therapist and occupational therapy assistant.	X	X
Demonstrates skill in evidence-based practice; makes informed practice decisions.	Incorporated into Evaluation/ Screening and Intervention sections.	X

Note. FWPE/OTS = Fieldwork Performance Evaluation for the Occupational Therapy Student; FWPE/OTAS = Fieldwork Performance Evaluation for the Occupational Therapy Assistant Student.

Table 10. Comparison of Evaluation/Screening Items on the *FWPE/OTS* and *FWPE/OTAS*

Item No. and Description *FWPE/OTS*		Item No. and Description *FWPE/OTAS*	
8	Articulates a clear, logical rationale.		
9	Selects relevant methods.		
13	Administers assessments in a uniform manner.	8	Establishes service competency in assessment methods.
10	Determines client's occupational profile and performance.	7	Under supervision and cooperation with the occupational therapist/occupational therapy assistant, gathers information.
11	Assesses client and contextual factors that support or hinder occupational performance.		
12	Obtains sufficient and necessary information from relevant sources.		
14	Adjusts/modifies the assessment procedures based on client's needs, behaviors, and culture.		
15	Interprets evaluation results to determine occupational performance strengths and challenges.	9	Assists with interpreting assessments in relation to the client's performance and goals in collaboration.
16	Establishes accurate plan based on evaluation results integrating multiple factors.	11	Develops client-centered and occupation-based goals in collaboration with the occupational therapist.
17	Documents results of the evaluation process in objective terms.	10	Reports results accurately.

Note. FWPE/OTS = Fieldwork Performance Evaluation for the Occupational Therapy Student; FWPE/OTAS = Fieldwork Performance Evaluation for the Occupational Therapy Assistant Student.

ation tasks. Any state licensure laws that dictate the roles and responsibilities of occupational therapists and occupational therapy assistants in practice always supersede AOTA guidelines. It is important to note that evaluation items on the *FWPE/OTAS* primarily focus on evaluating and reporting the results of daily interventions. However, in some settings, occupational therapy assistant students may assist with gathering initial information after service competency is established. Examples of objectives that clarify the expectations of occupational therapy assistant students' abilities in this section include

- After establishing service competency, accurately administers the Allen Cognitive Level Test.
- Efficiently assesses ADL using guided observations of all clients.
- Submits weekly revisions to client goals during supervision meeting with the occupational therapist.

Occupational therapy students are required to demonstrate competency in all aspects of the evaluation process, including

- Stating how and why a specific approach to the evaluation process is being used (Item 8, Rationale).
- Accurately gathering information related to the client's occupational profile (who he or she is, his or her interests, values, and goals, and patterns of daily life) and occupational performance (the actual ability to perform), as well as the client factors (called *components* in *Uniform Terminology III*) and context (called *environment* in *Uniform Terminology III*) (Items 10 and 11) (AOTA, 1994).
- Selecting, accurately using, and adjusting methods and tools when gathering information (Items 9, 12, and 13).
- Interpreting the data from an occupational therapy perspective (summarizing what the client can or cannot do, along with the factors that either support or hinder performance) to plan interventions that reflect an understanding of multiple factors. (This is an example of how a student's abili-

ty to integrate and bring information together can be assessed.) (Items 15 and 16)

- Documenting the evaluation in a way that demonstrates progress and shows the efficacy of occupational therapy (Item 17).

Site-specific objectives for occupational therapy students might address (a) specific assessments used, (b) types of assessment methods, (c) how goals and plans are written, or (d) some combination of these. For example, for the *FWPE/OTS* item Administers Assessments, site-specific objectives are written to reflect the essential skills required of occupational therapists in the facility. If one works in a hospital setting where the Functional Independence Measure™ (Hamilton, Granager, Sherwin, Zielezny, & Tashman, 1987) is routinely scored by occupational therapists, then a specific objective would be developed to reflect the student's proficiency in administering this specific assessment. In a community mental health setting, where the major evaluation method used is observation, an objective would

be written that clearly communicates to students that proficiency in observation is an essential skill that must be developed.

Intervention. The items in the Intervention section address skills used to deliver occupational therapy services, including selecting, implementing, and modifying services. Table 11 provides a comparison of the Intervention items on the *FWPE/OTS* and *FWPE/OTAS* and delineates the roles and responsibilities of each practitioner. Again, as stated under the Evaluation/Screening section, occupational therapy assistant students establish service competency and work in collaboration with occupational therapists when planning and modifying interventions.

Throughout the items in this section there is a clear emphasis on occupation-based and client-centered practice. The intent is to assist fieldwork educators and students in understanding the competencies needed to reflect readiness to practice as entry-level occupational therapists or occupational therapy assistants. Occupa-

Table 11. Comparison of Intervention Items on the *FWPE/OTS* and the *FWPE/OTAS*

Item No. and Description *FWPE/OTS*		Item No. and Description *FWPE/OTAS*	
18	Articulates clear rationale for the intervention process.		
19	Utilizes evidence to make informed intervention decisions.		
20	Chooses occupations that motivate and challenge clients.	12	In collaboration, establishes client-centered, occupation-based methods and duration and frequency of interventions.
21	Selects relevant occupations to facilitate clients meeting goals.	13	Selects and sequences interventions that promote engagement in occupations.
22	Implements intervention plans that are client-centered.	14	Implements occupation-based intervention in collaboration.
23	Implements interventions that are occupation-based.		
24	Modifies task approach, occupations, and the environment to maximize client performance.	15	Grades activities to motivate and challenge clients to facilitate progress.
		16	Effectively interacts with clients to facilitate accomplishment of established goals.
25	Updates, modifies, or terminates the intervention plan.	17	Monitors the clients' status to update, change, or terminate intervention plan in collaboration with the occupational therapist.
26	Documents client's response in a way that demonstrates efficacy of interventions.		

Note. FWPE/OTS = Fieldwork Performance Evaluation for the Occupational Therapy Student; FWPE/OTAS = Fieldwork Performance Evaluation for the Occupational Therapy Assistant Student.

tion is the domain of concern and the therapeutic medium of occupational therapy, and therefore students' abilities to promote engagement in occupation and to use occupation effectively in delivering services is an important competency to demonstrate. The content of site-specific objectives will communicate (a) the specific focus of occupation (e.g., in an acute setting the focus may be on basic self-care activities, whereas in a community setting the focus may be on work-related activities) and (b) the specific interventions (e.g., educates caregivers, implements group activities, fabricates splints, facilitates neuromuscular re-education) or intervention approaches (e.g., plans and implements interventions from the Model of Human Occupation and the Life Style Performance Model) in which students need to demonstrate competency for entry-level practice in a particular setting.

Management of occupational therapy services. The Management of Occupational Therapy Services section is found only in the *FWPE/OTS*. The five items address entry-level knowledge and skills related to funding and cost issues, supervision of occupational therapy and nonoccupational therapy personnel, and timeliness and volume of work. For occupational therapy assistant students, behaviors such as time management and volume of work are incorporated into items found in the Professional Behaviors section.

Items 27 and 28 address the roles and responsibilities of occupational therapists working with other occupational therapy personnel (occupational therapy assistants and occupational therapy aides). Item 27 addresses the ability of occupational therapy students to practice or discuss how to assign appropriate responsibilities to occupational therapy assistants or occupational therapy aides. Item 28 addresses the ability of students to practice or discuss how to collaborate with occupational therapy assistants. The task force recognizes that not all sites employ occupational therapy assistants or occupational therapy aides; thus, competency can be demonstrated through practice or discussion. These items are included because occupational therapy students are to be prepared, at entry-level, to supervise and work in cooperation with occupational therapy assistants (ACOTE, 1999a). Fieldwork is a natural learning environment in which to begin to gather this knowledge and skill. Discussion or practice in each fieldwork setting will help occupational therapy students generalize knowledge and skills and be prepared

for entry-level practice. When a fieldwork site does not employ occupational therapy assistants or occupational therapy aides, the objectives will clarify how students will demonstrate their knowledge. For example, specific objectives could include the following:

- Students discuss how to create and maintain a collaborative relationship with occupational therapy assistants.
- Students explain the duties of occupational therapists and occupational therapy assistants in the school system.
- During the midterm evaluation meetings, students describe to fieldwork educators the roles of occupational therapy assistants.
- After site visits, students differentiate roles of occupational therapy assistants and occupational therapists during the occupational therapy process.

Communication. Items in the Communication section on evaluation forms of both the *FWPE/OTS* and the *FWPE/OTAS* address competencies related to effective communication (verbal and nonverbal) and clear, accurate documentation (see Table 12). In addition, the *FWPE/OTS* includes two additional items related specifically to documenting (a) the results of the evaluation in an objective manner (Item 17) and (b) the client's response to services in a manner that demonstrates the efficacy of interventions (Item 26). Occupational therapists and occupational therapy assistants communicate information about occupational therapy services to various recipients both verbally and in writing. For both occupational therapy and occupational therapy assistant students, writing is required to be clear and accurate according to site requirements, as well as legible, with correct spelling, punctuation, and grammar. Developing site-specific objectives allows fieldwork educators to guide and assess students' abilities to produce documentation that reflects the specific language and requirements required at sites.

Professional behaviors. Items in the Professional Behaviors section address basic work skills and behaviors required of professionals, such as time management, respect for diversity, and interpersonal responsibilities for effective performance of job duties. The expectations for occupational therapy and occupational therapy assistant students are very similar. Many of these items are familiar to those who have used the previous evaluations, with one exception: cultural compe-

Table 12. Comparison of Communication Items on the *FWPE/OTS* and *FWPE/OTAS*

Item No. and Description *FWPE/OTS*	Item No. and Description *FWPE/OTAS*
32 Communicates verbally and nonverbally with clients and others.	18 Communicates verbally and nonverbally with clients and others.
33 Produces clear and accurate documentation according to site requirements.	19 Produces clear and accurate documentation according to site requirements. All writing is legible; uses proper spelling, punctuation, and grammar.
34 All writing is legible; uses proper spelling, punctuation, and grammar.	
35 Uses language appropriate to the recipient of the information, including, but not limited to, funding agencies and regulatory agencies.	

Note. FWPE/OTS = Fieldwork Performance Evaluation for the Occupational Therapy Student; FWPE/OTAS = Fieldwork Performance Evaluation for the Occupational Therapy Assistant Student.

tence. Students are required to demonstrate respect for the diversity of others, including but not limited to sociocultural, socioeconomic, spiritual, and lifestyle choices. The ability to work with and respect others is an important competency that recently has received greater attention in the profession. In addition, fieldwork educators often report this is an area of concern for some students and wanted a way to address this important area.

In summary, although the items on the *FWPE/OTS* and the *FWPE/OTAS* are conceptualized in concert with the occupational therapy process and reasoning used throughout the process, the items reflect the delineation of roles and responsibilities of occupational therapists and occupational therapy assistants.

Scoring Student Performance

Student competency develops over time. Therefore, the *FWPEs* are designed to measure change in performance from midterm to the final evaluation. Two features of the *FWPEs* help fieldwork educators in measuring the development of competency over time: (a) the rating scale and (b) the midterm and final scores. Following a review of each feature, general guidelines for scoring performance are discussed.

Rating Scale

The *FWPEs* share the same 4-point rating scale. Descriptors of the 4-point rating include both (a) a statement about the quality of students' performance

and (b) a description of when or how often the ratings might be used (see Exhibit 2). Through review of past fieldwork evaluations, and the results of the three pilot studies, it was found that using the rating scale accurately is a common problem. Fieldwork educators have a tendency to inflate students' scores. Also, if the rating scale is not used as designed, the ability of the evaluations to measure whether students are ready for entry-level practice is diminished. Therefore, each definition provides a point of reference when determining students' scores. This assists fieldwork educators in rating

Exhibit 2. Rating Scales for the *FWPE/OTS* and the *FWPE/OTAS*

4—Exceeds Standards: Performance is highly skilled and self-initiated. This rating is **rarely given** and **would represent the top 5% of all the students** you have supervised.

3—Meets Standards: Performance is consistent with **entry-level** practice. This rating is **infrequently given at midterm** and is a **strong rating at final**.

2—Needs Improvement: Performance **is progressing but** still needs improvement for entry-level practice. This is a **realistic rating of performance at midterm,** and some ratings of 2 may be reasonable at the final.

1—Unsatisfactory: Performance is **below standards** and requires development for entry-level practice. This rating is given when **there is a concern about performance.**

the competencies required for entry-level practice versus performance above entry-level practice.

It is important to remember that the rating scale is a 4-point scale; it is not designed to reflect a grade. If academic programs must give a grade for fieldwork, then it is up to the program to determine the grading strategy/configuration. Academic fieldwork coordinators (AFWCs) need to educate students on the fact that fieldwork experiences are "graded" using a different grading system than the traditional "A, B, C" grading system found in college/university systems. When students first come to the site, fieldwork educators are encouraged to review not only the *FWPE* items and objectives but also the rating scale that will be used.

Midterm and Final Scores

Students' performance is expected to develop over time; therefore, midterm and final scores will be different. Midterm and final cutoff scores, provided on the evaluation forms, assist students and fieldwork educators in assessing students' progress toward entry-level competence (see Table 13). Whether assessing performance at midterm or at the final, the point of reference remains the expectation for what students need to do by the end of the fieldwork to demonstrate entry-level competencies for specific fieldwork sites. Therefore, by providing minimum midterm requirements, both students and fieldwork educators know that at midterm students are performing satisfactorily. As well, having different minimum requirements for the midterm and the final reflects the fact that competency develops over time, and student performance needs to continue to develop beyond midterm to reach the established final competencies. For example, if a student "meets standards" across most items at midterm, fieldwork educators are in essence saying that the student is ready for practice and could stop the fieldwork rotation at this time. Preliminary midterm and final cutoff scores were determined through the pilot studies (see chapter 3 for more details). As long as students are performing satisfactorily and are meeting at least the minimum requirements, fieldwork educators may not be tempted to inflate students' ratings.

In addition, fieldwork educators and students need to realize that the *FWPE* items reflect a continuum of competencies that range from easier-to-reach items to harder-to-reach items. Therefore, students are not expected to score the same across all items whether at midterm or final. Table 4 on page 13 for the *FWPE/OTAS* and Table 6 on page 17 for the *FWPE/OTS* identify the continuum of easy to hard items. Referring back to these tables allows the fieldwork educator to compare students' patterns of performance with the expected pattern identified in the pilot studies. The *FWPEs* were designed so that the easier-to-reach competency items are more likely to be reached by all students, and the more competent the student is, the more likely it is that he or she will reach competency on easy-to-reach as well as hard-to-reach competency items. (See chapter 3 for more details.) For example, if a student scores a 1 and a 2 on safety and work behaviors (easier-to-reach competencies) but scores a 3 and a 4 on adjusting assessment procedures or intervention plans (harder-to-reach competencies), then the fieldwork educator should stop and reflect on what might be causing this pattern of performance, which is different than expected.

Table 13. Midterm and Final Cutoff Scores on the *FWPEs*

Overall Midterm Scores	FWPE/OTS	FWPE/OTAS
Satisfactory performance	90 points and above	54 points and above
Unsatisfactory performance	89 points and below	53 points and below

Overall Final Scores	FWPE/OTS	FWPE/OTAS
Pass	122 points and above	70 points and above
Not pass	121 points and below	69 points and below

Note. FWPE/OTS = Fieldwork Performance Evaluation for the Occupational Therapy Student; FWPE/OTAS = Fieldwork Performance Evaluation for the Occupational Therapy Assistant Student.

Guidelines for Scoring Student Performance

The evaluation forms are intended to be completed by both students and fieldwork educators separately, so that both parties bring their perspective and assessment together during the midterm and final reviews. Engagement in self-reflection and self-assessment is part of increasing one's competence and growth as a professional (Parham, 1987).

As stated earlier, developing objectives assists fieldwork educators in clarifying the expectations of students at the sites and not only improves the accuracy of scoring but also makes rating students' performance easier.

Each item must be scored; there are no "not applicable" items. If fieldwork educators determine that an item does not "fit" in a particular setting, then site-specific objectives will indicate how students will demonstrate abilities related to that item.

Students must pass all items in the Fundamentals of Practice section, earning a 3 or above at the final evaluation. Although the guidelines for the *FWPEs* do not state that students must pass each of these items at midterm, in most settings the expectation, even before midterm, is ethical and safe practice. Therefore, lack of attention to safety issues or unethical practice at any time can be grounds for failing fieldwork. Each fieldwork site may set or clarify higher standards and expectations based on what is required for entry-level practice in the setting. In the beginning of the fieldwork rotation, the expectations for acceptable behaviors need to be clearly stated; this can be done with site-specific objectives. If students are not passing these items at midterm, fieldwork educators should give clear, objective written feedback to ensure that students know what behaviors they need to demonstrate to pass the fieldwork at the final. In addition, AFWCs should be notified and involved any time there are concerns with student performance. If, at the time of the final, a student is not passing all three items, the fieldwork educator still must complete the entire evaluation to give the student feedback about his or her performance, even though he or she will not pass the fieldwork rotation.

At both the midterm and final evaluations the fieldwork educator rates each item and provides comments for each section. He or she then transfers midterm and final ratings to the Performance Rating Summary Sheet and compares overall midterm and final scores to the cutoff scales provided to determine whether students' performance meets the minimum requirements.

The *FWPEs* have a twofold purpose: (a) to measure entry-level competence rather than measuring the degrees of performance above entry-level and (b) to provide feedback to students about their performance over time. Readers are encouraged to read through the cases provided in chapter 5 to gain further knowledge of how to accurately use the rating scale.

Practical Applications of the Fieldwork Performance Evaluation Forms

This chapter provides case scenarios to illustrate how to use the *FWPEs*. When using the evaluation forms, fieldwork educators should keep in mind the context of the fieldwork rotation when determining how to rate entry-level competency. Knowledge, skills, and abilities required of occupational therapists and occupational therapy assistants differ from setting to setting; therefore, what is considered entry-level varies from facility to facility. The specific expectations for each site are reflected in the site-specific objectives written to supplement the items on the *FWPEs*.

The four case scenarios illustrate how (a) the evaluation forms can be individualized to fit various settings, (b) student performance is rated, and (c) the space for comments is used to provide clear feedback and guidance at midterm. It is important to remember that fieldwork educators rate student performance over time, rather than according to a single incident, which is difficult to illustrate with a written case scenario. Whether at midterm or final, fieldwork educators are comparing students' performance to the roles and responsibilities of entry-level occupational therapists or occupational therapy assistants in the setting; thus, midterm ratings will not be as high as the final ratings, and most students will not meet standards on most items at midterm.

Each case scenario begins with a brief description of the fieldwork setting and performance expectations (site-specific objectives written to accompany the *FWPE* items) of the student by the end of the fieldwork rotation. Brief snapshots of students' performance during fieldwork are broken into segments to reflect midterm or final performance (or both). In the first two case scenarios a few sections of the *FWPEs* are presented to illustrate ratings and comments. Midterm comments illustrate how the comment section is used to guide and clarify what the student needs to do to obtain a "meets standards" rating at the final. In the second two case scenarios, performance ratings and rationales for ratings are discussed.

Case 1: Carrie—
Occupational Therapy Student in Community Setting

Community Connections is a community-based program that provides a variety of services and education activities, including vocational assessment, job placement, and ongoing case management and support to enhance community living for participants with brain injuries. Some of the knowledge, skills, and abilities that occupational therapy Level II fieldwork students are expected to demonstrate include the following:

- Communicating to a variety of participants and potential job placement sites what occupational therapy is in language that is understandable to the recipients.
- Routinely selecting, administering, and interpreting assessments based on the clients' presenting condition and the pragmatics of the situation. This includes
  - using client-centered assessments,
  - accurately completing home and work site assessments, and
  - gathering accurate and complete information through telephone interviews.
- Writing narrative reports that clearly identify the participants' occupational performance strengths and challenges.
- Using experiential activities when delivering community presentations.

Carrie's performance, Weeks 1–6. During the first 3 weeks, Carrie and her supervisor assisted participants in identifying job preferences, setting up and engaging in interviews, and establishing daily routines to support engagement in homemaking activities.

By Week 4, Carrie took over primary responsibility in planning and carrying out interventions with two participants, Sally and Joe. Carrie was observed to consistently ask participants what they wanted to be doing and often did what the participants wanted to be doing without offering her input or suggestions to guide intervention. The activities participants identified helped them reach their desired outcomes, but the activities were not always sequenced in a manner that promoted reaching the outcome directly or efficiently. For example, Joe attended a preliminary job placement assessment that did not go as planned. Carrie chose the work environment based solely on Joe's interests and did not take into consideration Joe's challenges (i.e., that he fatigues quickly when standing and working for more than 1 hour at a time). The potential employment site was disappointed because they thought Joe would be working for them immediately. Talking with her supervisor, Carrie realized that she did not attempt to modify the situation. After discussing things with her supervisor, Carrie began to recognize ways to update Joe's plan.

During Week 5, Carrie opened a new case. On their first visit at the Community Connections office, Carrie shared with Eric (the new participant) and his family the mission and philosophy of the organization. Describing the information from the Community Connections Web site about services provided, Carrie proceeded to state she would help Eric engage in "occupations Eric finds meaningful." Eric quickly responded that he was enthusiastic, because he had "always wanted to start his own business." After the meeting, Carrie discussed with her fieldwork educator that she wanted to spend time with Eric in his home, as well as accompanying him as he traveled around the community using the bus and interacting with others, to observe him engaging in both familiar and unfamiliar activities. Carrie expressed that this would allow her to get a better feel for what Eric was able to do and that these activities would fall under acceptable occupational therapy evaluation and intervention for reimbursement from vocational rehabilitation. During the midterm review, Carrie accurately talked about the general role of occupational therapy assistants across settings.

Refer to Figure 9 to see how Carrie's supervisor scored her midterm performance. Note how the comments support the ratings given and provide Carrie feedback on areas in which she needs to continue to improve.

Carrie's performance, Weeks 7–12. During the next 6 weeks, Carrie continued to work with her assigned participants, helped give a presentation to a local head injury support group, and wrote letters seeking further funding for her assigned participants. The letters that she wrote resulted in an increase in funds for two of her

Figure 9. Selected Items From Carrie's *FWPE/OTS*

RATING SCALE FOR THE STUDENT PERFORMANCE

4—Exceeds Standards: Performance is highly skilled and self-initiated. This rating is **rarely given** and **would represent the top 5% of all the students** you have supervised.

3—Meets Standards: Performance is consistent with **entry-level** practice. This rating is **infrequently given at midterm** and is a **strong rating at final**.

2—Needs Improvement: Performance is **progressing but** still needs improvement for entry-level practice. This is a **realistic rating of performance at midterm,** and some ratings of 2 may be reasonable at the final.

1—Unsatisfactory: Performance is **below standards** and requires development for entry-level practice. This rating is given when **there is a concern about performance.**

II. BASIC TENETS

4. Clearly and confidently **articulates the values and beliefs** of the occupational therapy profession to clients, families, significant others, colleagues, service providers, and the public.

Midterm	1	**2**	3	4
Final	1	2	**3**	4

7. **Collaborates with** client, family, and significant others throughout the occupational therapy process.

Midterm	**1**	2	3	4
Final	1	2	**3**	4

Comments on strengths and areas for improvement:

• **Midterm** Shares accurate information about organization and occupational therapy. Continue to work on your clarity of explaining what occupational therapy is. Continue to work on individualizing the information, using terms and language that the recipients will understand. Engages participants in discussions, but process is not collaborative. Collaborate with others by sharing your ideas with the client and together making decisions.

• **Final** Nice growth and change in being able to explain occupational therapy to a variety of different people. You have learned how to bring your perspective and the participant's perspective together in planning and carrying out services. *(Continued)*

assigned participants. In the letters, Carrie effectively used research study results to support her rationale for requesting additional funds to purchase adaptive equipment.

Carrie had been trying to locate potential employment opportunities for Sally. Carrie shared with her

Figure 9. Continued

III. EVALUATION AND SCREENING

8. **Articulates a clear and logical rationale** for the evaluation process.

Midterm	1	**2**	3	4
Final	1	2	**3**	4

16 **Establishes an accurate and appropriate plan** based on the evaluation results, through integrating multiple factors such as client's priorities, context(s), theories, and evidence-based practice.

Midterm	1	**2**	3	4
Final	1	2	**3**	4

Comments on strengths and areas for improvement:

• **Midterm** Shares beginning rationale for choice of activities to observe with Eric. Planned job assessment for Joe based only on participant's priorities, not other factors. Continue to establish plans that address participant's abilities and available resources/opportunities in the community.

• **Final** Your ability to assess and re-assess client performance during job assessments illustrates how you can now identify, interpret, and plan for adjustments during services. Nice job with working with Sally, integrating her priorities with the work site demands and occupational therapy theory. You also effectively used evidence-based research to support your rationale in obtaining additional funding. Your ability to clearly explain your reasons for selecting approaches will support you, no matter what setting you decide to work in.

IV. INTERVENTION

21. **Selects relevant occupations** to facilitate clients meeting established goals.

Midterm	1	**2**	3	4
Final	1	2	**3**	4

25. **Updates, modifies or terminates intervention plan** based on careful monitoring of the client's status.

Midterm	**1**	2	3	4
Final	1	2	**3**	4

Comments on strengths and areas for improvement:

• **Midterm** Strong ability to select activities participants want to engage in. Participants appear invested in services (which does not always happen), but you are not selecting activities effectively to help reach the goals. Continue to think about what may be the best activities and sequence of activities to assist participants in meeting the overall outcome established. Be prepared to discuss observations you are making that lead to your decisions to modify or change plans.

• **Final** You now have a strong ability to select and use activities effectively to help participants meet their goals. In addition, you have shown considerable growth in updating plans. Continue to work on this in your next fieldwork.

V. MANAGEMENT OF OCCUPATIONAL THERAPY SERVICES

27. **Demonstrates through practice or discussion the ability to assign** appropriate responsibilities to the occupational therapy assistant and occupational therapy aide.

Midterm	1	**2**	3	4
Final	1	2	**3**	4

29. **Demonstrates understanding of the costs and funding** related to occupational therapy services at this site.

Midterm	1	**2**	3	4
Final	1	2	3	**4**

Comments on strengths and areas for improvement:

• **Midterm** Discussed general role of the occupational therapy assistant across settings. Prior to final evaluation, be prepared to discuss specific tasks of your caseload you would assign to an occupational therapy assistant. Also in discussion showed beginning knowledge of voc[ational] rehab. Begin to identify and seek out community resources for funding issues, and consider information on funding when you are prioritizing services.

• **Final** Your understanding of issues related to voc[ational] rehab funding has supported your ability to prioritize how you spend time with your participants. Letters written to seek funding for several participants to support the continuation of employment support were very effective.

fieldwork educator that she had talked with Sally's vocational rehabilitation case manager to clarify funding and had made several telephone calls to potential sites, two of which agreed to have Sally come and work for 1 hour in the morning. The job tasks entailed doing preparatory work. Through talking with Carrie, the fieldwork educator determined that Carrie had gathered sufficient information about the job/task requirements at the two sites and that she had thought through ways she could grade the activity for Sally to be able to complete the required tasks in the allotted time. After completion of the first site visit with Sally, Carrie reported back that she had anticipated Sally's needs for simplifying the environment and the task but had not anticipated how difficult it would be for Sally to stand while using both hands to wash and chop vegetables. Carrie stated she guided Sally through problem-solving the situation, and together they identified additional aspects to think about when visiting the next site. When her fieldwork educator asked her what she considered when making changes to the plan, Carrie identified the following: Sally's needs, the expectations of the work site, and biomechanical principles.

Both during and after the presentation that Carrie and her fieldwork educator gave to the head injury support group, Carrie interacted with several families and service providers, discussing how occupational therapy can assist people who have sustained a head injury. During each interaction, Carrie used different wording and varied examples to promote understanding of concepts. In the last week, during weekly supervision, Carrie talked about which of the tasks she was doing would be appropriate to assign to an occupational therapy assistant. Carrie's knowledge was accurate.

Case 2: Paula—
Occupational Therapy Assistant Student in
Community Mental Health Group Home

Mountain Vista is a group home for people with chronic mental health issues that provides a supervised setting before transition into less-restrictive living arrangements. Most of the residents subsist on social security income. Both one-to-one and group interventions are provided in a therapeutic milieu. Some of the knowledge, skills, and abilities that occupational therapy assistant Level II fieldwork students are expected to demonstrate include the following:

- Consistently following the home's policies and procedures for creating and maintaining a therapeutic milieu (during all activities, in house, and in the community).
- Consistently being a strong role model for effective communication through all interactions with residents and staff.
- Locating, effectively using, and initiating discussion about resources being used to guide own learning.
- Assisting with development and implementation of at least one new programming idea.
- Effectively leading daily groups, ensuring that res-

idents' individual goals are being addressed.
- Writing daily objective notes, reflecting residents' abilities, adhering to the home's guidelines.

Paula's performance, Weeks 1–4. Paula has two supervisors: the day program coordinator, who has a background in human development and psychology, and an occupational therapist, who works as a case manager for the county mental health system.

From the first day, Paula willingly assisted with the daily setup of group activities and the cleanup of the common living areas and staff lounge. She did these tasks with the group home staff for the first week but then suggested to the day program coordinator that she incorporate the group home residents in these activities. Paula clearly followed the home's protocol for initiating or changing daily programming. Paula discussed her ideas with both of her supervisors prior to initiating them. She identified which residents would be appropriate to engage in the cleaning activities but required a lot of guidance in deciding which activities each resident could engage in. As Paula began to facilitate residents' involvement, she gave three- to four-step directions to the residents and was confused and frustrated when the residents did not follow her directions. In their weekly supervisory meeting, Paula and her supervisors discussed this situation. After responding to several questions posed by the occupational therapy supervisor, Paula understood and saw how the residents' cognitive abilities were affecting their performance. Paula used her textbooks to research cognitive impairments and created a list of various intervention strategies to use to adapt the activities for successful performance. Over the next couple of weeks, Paula continued to require meetings with her on-site supervisor each day to help her grade the activities.

During weekly supervision, Paula talked about how she was still feeling awkward with interacting with some of the residents, particularly those who had no affect and those who were very talkative. Paula's on-site supervisor agreed with Paula's assessment of her interactions and provided some suggestions for improvement.

During Week 4, Paula began coleading the daily groups, including noon meal preparations with the group home staff. The staff reported that Paula was always prepared and willing to help out but that she needed to continue to work on her interactions with the residents. In particular, there was a concern that Paula

Figure 10. Selected Items From Paula's *FWPE/OTAS*

I. FUNDAMENTALS OF PRACTICE

1. **Ethics:** Adheres consistently to the AOTA Code of Ethics and site's policies and procedures.

Midterm	1	2	**3**	4
Final	1	2	**3**	4

2. **Safety:** Adheres consistently to safety regulations. Anticipates potentially hazardous situations and takes steps to prevent accidents.

Midterm	1	**2**	3	4
Final	1	2	**3**	4

3. **Safety:** Uses sound judgment in regard to safety of self and others during all fieldwork-related activities.

Midterm	1	**2**	3	4
Final	1	2	**3**	4

Comments on strengths and areas for improvement

• **Midterm** You have demonstrated good awareness of policies and procedures at the home, and beginning insight into safety and judgment issues. Continue to pay attention to these important issues in this setting.

• **Final** You have made some nice gains in this area.

IV. INTERVENTION

12. **Plans Intervention:** In collaboration with the occupational therapist, establishes methods, duration, and frequency of interventions that are client-centered and occupation-based. Intervention plans reflect context of setting.

Midterm	1	**2**	3	4
Final	1	2	**3**	4

14. **Implements Intervention:** Implements occupation-based interventions effectively in collaboration with clients, families, significant others, and service providers.

Midterm	1	**2**	3	4
Final	1	2	**3**	4

15. **Activity Analysis:** Grades activities to motivate and challenge clients in order to facilitate progress.

Midterm	**1**	2	3	4
Final	1	2	**3**	4

16. **Therapeutic Use of Self:** Effectively interacts with clients to facilitate accomplishment of established goals.

Midterm	**1**	2	3	4
Final	1	**2**	3	4

Comments on strengths and areas for improvement

• **Midterm** With assistance, you are able to plan and carry out interventions. You have some great ideas. With continued practice, you will be an effective service provider. Focus efforts on learning how to grade and adapt interventions. You have made improvement with use of self, but need to focus on this area. This is a tough setting, but it is critical to be effective.

• **Final** You have shown great improvements in the area of providing interventions, particularly with leading groups and grading activities. You need to continue to work on effective interactions, particularly learning to set boundaries with inappropriate comments from clients.

V. COMMUNICATION

19. **Written Communication:** Produces clear and accurate documentation according to site requirements. All writing is legible, using proper spelling, punctuation, and grammar.

Midterm	1	**2**	3	4
Final	1	2	**3**	4

Comments on strengths and areas for improvement

• **Midterm** You have made good progress on making notes more objective. Continue to work on conciseness.

• **Final** Your documentation is very effective. Your notes clearly describe the residents' skills and abilities to engage in occupations. Nice job!

VI. PROFESSIONAL BEHAVIORS

20. **Self-Responsibility:** Takes responsibility for attaining professional competence by seeking out learning opportunities and interactions with supervisor(s) and others.

Midterm	1	2	**3**	4
Final	1	2	**3**	4

22. **Work Behaviors:** Demonstrates consistent work behaviors including initiative, preparedness, dependability, and work site maintenance

Midterm	1	2	**3**	4
Final	1	2	3	**4**

25. **Cultural Competence:** Demonstrates respect for diversity factors of others including but not limited to sociocultural, socioeconomic, spiritual, and lifestyle choices.

Midterm	1	**2**	3	4
Final	1	2	**3**	4

Comments on strengths and areas for improvement

• **Midterm** From Day 1 you have taken responsibility for your own learning and have been an asset here at the home. Always reliable. However you have a tendency to expect residents to share your same values/preferences (meal prep[aration]). Work to be more aware of differences, and demonstrate an ability to incorporate these factors in your services.

• **Final** Nice growth in the area of being aware of and working with cultural differences. If we had a job opening I would love to have you join us! Great worker, independent, and clearly takes responsibility for own learning.

needed to learn to respect residents' preferences and not force her values on them. Several times Paula had been observed trying to convince the residents that they should plan and prepare vegetarian meals (this was Paula's preference, not the residents'). In addition, the recipes she brought for residents to select from often required expensive gourmet items.

Paula began writing notes during her second week of her fieldwork. Her notes were quite lengthy and descriptive, although they usually focused on how the clients were feeling rather than on their skills and abilities to engage in purposeful activity/occupations. By Week 4, Paula's notes had improved; they now focused on the clients' skills and abilities, although they were still too lengthy.

Paula's performance, Weeks 5–8. Paula continued to facilitate residents' engagement in keeping the common living areas clean and organized and required less direction for daily grading and adapting the activities.

Paula has been assisting the day staff in providing guidance with the noon meal preparations and consistently wrote clear objectives and concise notes indicating the residents' engagement in task roles. During Week 5, Paula initiated taking over the primary responsibilities of helping the residents plan, prepare, and clean up lunch. Paula developed a system in which the residents meet on Monday morning to select menus, plan and complete grocery shopping, and develop the schedule for rotating cooking and cleaning responsibilities. Paula expanded recipe selections to include residents' preferences and worked with the residents on how to plan and buy groceries within a given budget. With the assistance of the day program coordinator, Paula easily and accurately matched tasks to residents' abilities to facilitate progress toward their weekly goals.

Paula has been leading the socialization group in which residents plan and carry out community outings. Fred is a new client who has joined the group recently. Fred talks excessively throughout the group sessions, and one day in particular he kept asking Paula about her chipped tooth. Throughout the group session, Fred kept up a stream of comments, complimenting Paula on her clothes and hair. After several unsuccessful attempts to redirect Fred, Paula decided to end the group early, as she did not feel anyone was gaining anything from the group. After the incident, Paula asked to talk with both of her supervisors to discuss the group dynamics. In talking the situation over with the occupational therapy supervisor, Paula discussed how she had learned how to engage clients who tend to be withdrawn but that she still struggles with how to redirect clients who lack self-control. The staff from the group home who attended community outings with Paula indicated that Paula consistently follows policies and procedures for activities outside the home. The staff also reported that, while Paula's interactions with residents have become more effective, she continues to struggle with clients who talk a lot. Paula's evaluation can be found in Figure 10.

Case 3: Brian— Occupational Therapy Student in Skilled Nursing Facility

Northern Manor is a long-term care facility with a skilled nursing staff that provides rehabilitation services for patients planning to return home or to assisted living. The facility is an accredited provider for Medicare and the Kaiser health maintenance organization. The typical length of stay is 2–6 weeks. Some of the knowledge, skills, and abilities that occupational therapy Level II fieldwork students are expected to demonstrate include the following:

- Explaining occupational therapy in layman's terms to family and residents.
- Gathering residents' occupational status through effective and efficient interviewing and objective observation of ADL and IADL.
- Accurately completing the Minimum Data Set forms.
- Effectively delivering occupation-based interventions in a timely manner.
- Effectively collaborating with other health care professionals.
- Maintaining 60% work productivity.

Brian's performance, Weeks 1–4 (12-week rotation). Brian has been working closely with his supervisor and her caseload. Brian is seeing three patients and has had the opportunity to complete portions of two initial evaluations. Recently, as Brian's supervisor reduced the amount of structure and constant supervision she was providing, several concerns emerged. The physical therapy staff expressed concerns that Brian is "always running over his scheduled time" and that patients are refusing to participate in occupational therapy because they do not see the purpose of the activities. Brian states that he recognizes how important it is to allow clients to be comfortable, so he spends more time trying to help them feel comfortable. He has not changed or updated any of the intervention ideas. After further discussion with Brian, his fieldwork educator discovers that Brian does not understand how to set up the activities to make them therapeutic or how to modify the activities.

During the latest evaluation, Brian spent 45 minutes with Mr. Jones, who was admitted with congestive heart failure. His past medical history includes chronic obstructive pulmonary disease and anxiety disorder. Brian spent the entire time visiting with Mr. Jones, who spoke about his life history, focusing most of his time on talking about how he met his wife 50 years ago. Brian stated that he wanted to be supportive of Mr. Jones, and so he decided to let Mr. Jones talk about his wife, because how they met seemed to be important to him. Later, Brian reported that he felt satisfied with the interview because he gathered the same information that the social worker did on her intake interview. That same afternoon, Brian's fieldwork educator assisted him in completing a performance and task analysis of toileting with Mr. Jones. Although Brian stated that monitoring vital signs would help him determine the extent to which cardiopulmonary function was affecting performance, Brian required significant assistance in gathering the information. Two weeks before, his supervisor demonstrated how to take vital signs and had Brian practice the techniques before working with the patient. Brian required significant help and was instructed to continue to practice these skills. The following week, during a conference with Mr. Jones's family, Brian's supervisor had to step in and help explain to the family why Mr. Jones had been engaging in card games during occupational therapy interventions.

At weekly rounds, Brian reported on the three patients he was seeing. He summarized the patients' goals for discharge but did not objectively share the progress they were making. After rounds, Brian frequently left his written notes, with patients' names and status, lying around in the patients' and families' dining room.

Brian's fieldwork educator has repeatedly met with him, providing him with direct, clear feedback about the importance of confidentiality and issues with safety and time management. Brian continues to say he is "working on it" and appreciates the input. Because of Brian's lack of progress even when given direct, concrete feedback, his fieldwork educator decided to use the *FWPE/OTS* at Week 4 to rate his performance (Table 14). This was done to set objectives that Brian must meet at midterm to continue his fieldwork rotation past midterm.

Brian is not passing fieldwork and is at great risk for not satisfactorily completing the experience. One would hope that the academic fieldwork coordinator has been involved, and specific objectives and timelines have been established. It is clear that Brian needs to demonstrate significant progress in 2 weeks, at midterm, or his fieldwork will be discontinued.

Case 4: Jill—
Occupational Therapy Assistant Student in Acute Psychiatric Hospital

Glen Haven Hospital is an acute-care psychiatric hospital. Its services focus on evaluating, stabilizing, and referring patients to community resources. Some of the knowledge, skills, and abilities that occupational therapy assistant Level II fieldwork students are expected to demonstrate include the following:

- Consistently following all safety guidelines.
- Efficiently setting up for daily occupational therapy groups.
- Effectively facilitating two occupational therapy groups a day.
- Accurately documenting patients' performance and behavior after occupational therapy groups and ward activities.
- Assisting with monitoring patient activities on and off the ward.
- Providing weekly activities on the ward.
- Accurately screening all incoming patients using the Allen Cognitive Level Test (ACL) and structured intake interview.

Jill's performance, Weeks 1–4 (8-week rotation). Jill's supervisor is the occupational therapy assistant on staff at the hospital. After her orientation to the hospital's policies and procedures, Jill began spending time on the ward and observing occupational therapy groups. Jill continued to take on more responsibilities and by Week 4 was setting up for all occupational therapy groups. Jill often would come in early or not take lunch so she could get the groups set up on time, because it seemed to take her longer than the time allotted. In addition, Jill was leading two low-functioning groups per week. During the craft group Jill was effectively monitoring patients' frustration tolerance for the activities and would step in and provide additional structure as needed. Jill was accurately selecting craft activities to use

Table 14. Selected Item Ratings and Rationales for Brian's Performance

Item	Rating	Rationale for the Rating
1. **Adheres to ethics...**	1	Despite feedback, Brian is not able to maintain confidentiality of patient information. He continues to leave notes in public spaces.
10. **Determines client's occupational profile...**	1	Ineffective interview methods used when attempting to gather Mr. Jones's occupational status. Does not gather the information, and does not keep the interview focused.
12. **Obtains sufficient and necessary information...**	1	Gathered same information that had already been gathered during social work intake. Did not gather sufficient and necessary information about Mr. Jones's occupational status.
13. **Administers assessments in uniform manner ...**	1	Even after demonstration and practice, is not able to accurately take vital signs. No carryover of learning noted.
14. **Adjusts/modifies the assessment procedures...**	1	Brian makes no attempt to modify the assessment procedures, even after discussion with supervisor.
22. **Implements intervention plans that are occupation-based.**	1	Even after 4 weeks of constant supervision and structure, Brian is still not able to use occupations effectively to help patients meet their goals.
24. **Modifies task approach, occupations, and the environment...**	1	Even after 4 weeks of constant supervision and structure, Brian is still not able to use occupations effectively to help patients meet their goals. Through discussion with Brian, it became evident that he did not know how to set up the activities, nor how to modify them.
32. **Clearly and effectively communicates verbally and nonverbally...**	1	Brian is not effective in his communication style with the patients as: (a) he is not able to direct the conversation to gather necessary information and (b) the patients do not understand the purpose of therapy. Brian also has not communicated well during weekly meetings.
38. **Responds constructively to feedback.**	1	Brian has not adjusted or modified his behavior following feedback from his supervisor.
40. **Demonstrates effective time management.**	1	Brian is ineffective with his time and is unable to manage his time with the patients. Have received complaints from other staff.

with patients; however, Jill had not begun to take the lead in the higher functioning groups yet, as she stated she wanted more time to observe. When questioned further, Jill reported that the higher functioning groups seemed to require more ability to monitor patients' performance and modify activities and that she was not comfortable with having so many patients at different functioning levels.

In Week 3, Jill planned activities for the patients on the ward. Jill brought in notes from school that gave suggestions for one-step simple activities. The majority of the patients engaged in the activities, but when Jill was sharing her ideas with her supervisor she stated, "I just used these because we had talked about them in class."

After observing her supervisor complete several intake screenings, Jill completed two with her supervisor present. After each one, Jill's supervisor reviewed the procedures and gave specific feedback on how to complete the ACL. Last week, Jill was unable to complete the ACL with a patient, and Jill asked her supervisor to complete the intake interview. After discussing the situation, both Jill and her supervisor agreed that much of her difficulty in completing the ACL is related to not following the standardized procedures, and in the intake interview Jill is not able to clearly share what the role of occupational therapy is in this facili-

Table 15. Selected Item Ratings and Rationales for Jill's Performance

Item	Rating	Rationale for the Rating
2. **Safety**	3	Jill consistently adheres to safety precautions both in the occupational therapy clinic and on the ward.
4. **Occupational Therapy Philosophy**	2	During intake interview, Jill had difficulty stating what occupational therapy is and talking about the role in this setting.
6. **Evidence-based Practice**	2	Jill used notes from her academic program to support her ideas for intervention, but has a weak understanding of how these ideas have guided her interactions/interventions.
7. **Gathers Data**	2	Jill is having difficulty obtaining the needed information to complete the screenings, but during group intervention is able to identify behaviors and actions to modify intervention.
8. **Administers Assessments**	1	Jill has not been able to establish service competency yet in administering the ACL or the structured intake interview.
13. **Selects Intervention**	2	Jill has been able to begin planning and making suggestions for appropriate group activities for the lower level groups, and she has also planned and selected an appropriate activity for the ward activities.
14. **Implements Intervention**	1	Jill has been leading the lower-functioning group twice a week, but has not attempted to lead the higher-functioning group. She will need to be able to run both groups, and also increase the number of times per week she is leading the groups.
17. **Modifies Intervention Plan**	2	Jill has been able to modify interventions both following completion of the daily groups and coming up with ideas for what to do next time. As well, during the groups, she has demonstrated her ability to adapt the activity to decrease the patient's frustration.
23. **Time Management**	2	Jill has determined a way to complete her assigned duties, but is not being able to efficiently complete set-up for groups in a timely manner.

ty. Patients keep stating that they don't need a job.

Several of the fieldwork educator's midterm ratings and rationale for the ratings for Jill are provided in Table 15.

Jill is making progress in developing basic competencies for the occupational therapy assistant student. She will need to continue to develop skills and abilities in many areas.

References

Accreditation Council for Occupational Therapy Education. (1999a). Standards for an accredited educational program for the occupational therapist. *American Journal of Occupational Therapy, 53,* 575–582.

Accreditation Council for Occupational Therapy Education. (1999b). Standards for an accredited educational program for the occupational therapy assistant. *American Journal of Occupational Therapy, 53,* 583–589.

American Occupational Therapy Association. (1983). *Fieldwork evaluation form for occupational therapy assistant students.* Rockville, MD: Author.

American Occupational Therapy Association. (1987). *Fieldwork evaluation form for the occupational therapist.* Rockville, MD: Author.

American Occupational Therapy Association. (1994). Uniform terminology for occupational therapy, third edition. *American Journal of Occupational Therapy, 48,* 1047–1059.

American Occupational Therapy Association. (1998). Standards of practice for occupational therapy. *American Journal of Occupational Therapy, 52,* 866–869.

American Occupational Therapy Association. (1999a). Glossary: Standards for an accredited educational program for the occupational therapist and occupational therapy assistant. *American Journal of Occupational Therapy, 53,* 590–591.

American Occupational Therapy Association. (1999b). Standards for an accredited educational program for the occupational therapist. *American Journal of Occupational Therapy, 53,* 575–582.

American Occupational Therapy Association. (1999c). Standards for an accredited educational program for the occupational therapy assistant. *American Journal of Occupational Therapy, 53,* 583–589.

American Occupational Therapy Association. (2000). Occupational therapy code of ethics. *American Journal of Occupational Therapy, 54,* 614–616.

American Occupational Therapy Association. (2002). Occupational therapy practice framework: Domain and process. *American Journal of Occupational Therapy, 56,* 606–639.

American Physical Therapy Association. (1997). *Physical therapist clinical performance instrument.* Alexandria, VA: Author.

American Speech–Language–Hearing Association. (1997). *Membership and certification handbook.* Rockville, MD: Author.

Andrich, D. (1988). *Rasch models for measurement.* Newbury Park, CA: Sage.

Bond, T., & Fox, C. (2001). *Applying the Rasch model: Fundamental measurement in the human sciences.* Hillsdale, NJ: Erlbaum.

Bonello, M. (2001). Fieldwork within the context of higher education: A literature review. *British Journal of Occupational Therapy, 64,* 93–99.

Bridge, C. E., & Twible, R. L. (1997). Clinical reasoning. In C. H. Christiansen & C. M. Baum (Eds.), *Occupational therapy: Enabling function and well-being* (2nd ed., pp. 159–179). Thorofare, NJ: Slack.

Christiansen, C. H., & Baum, C. M. (1997). Person–environment occupational performance. In C. H. Christiansen & C. M. Baum (Eds.), *Occupational therapy: Enabling function and well-being* (2nd ed., pp. 47–70). Thorofare, NJ: Slack.

Commission on Education of the American Occupational Therapy Association. (1994). *Guide to fieldwork education.* Rockville, MD: American Occupational Therapy Association.

Cooper, R. G., & Crist, P. A. (1988). Field test analysis and reliability of the fieldwork evaluation for the occupational therapist. *Occupational Therapy Journal of Research, 8,* 369–379.

Coster, W., Denney, T., Haltiwanger, J., & Haley, S. (1998). *School function assessment.* San Antonio, TX: Psychological Corporation.

Creek, J. (1997). Approaches to practice. In J. Creek (Ed.), *Occupational therapy and mental health* (pp. 71–89). New York: Churchill Livingstone.

Crist, P. A., & Cooper, R. G. (1988). Evaluating clinical competence with the new fieldwork evaluation. *American Journal of Occupational Therapy, 42,* 771–773.

Crocker, L. M., Muthard, J. E., Slaymaker, J. E., & Samson, L. (1975). A performance rating scale for evaluating clinical competence of occupational therapy students. *American Journal of Occupational Therapy, 29,* 81–86.

Culler, K. (1991). Assessment of OT student performance. In *Self-paced instruction for clinical education and supervision* (pp. 241–286). Rockville, MD: American Occupational Therapy Association.

Ernest, M., & Polatajko, H. J. (1986). Performance evaluation of occupational therapy students: A validity study. *Canadian Journal of Occupational Therapy, 53,* 265–271.

Fearing, V. G., & Clark, J. (Eds.). (2000). *Individuals in context: A practical guide to client-centered practice.* Thorofare, NJ: Slack.

Fisher, A. G. (2001). *Assessment of motor and process skills* (4th ed.). Fort Collins, CO: Three Star Press.

Fisher, A. G., Bryze, K. A., Granger, C. V., Haley, S. M., Hamilton, B. B., Heinemann, A. W., Puderbaugh, J. K., Linacre, J. M., Ludlow, L. H., McCabe, M. A., & Wright, B. D. (1994). Applications of conjoint measurement to the development of functional assessments. *International Journal of Educational Research, 21,* 579–593.

Fisher, W. P. (1993). Measurement-related problems in functional assessment. *American Journal of Occupational Therapy, 47,* 331–338.

Hager, P., & Gonczi, A. (1996). What is competence? *Medical Teacher, 18*(1), 15–18.

Haley, S. M., & Ludlow, L. H. (1992). Applicability of the hierarchical scales of the Tufts Assessment of Motor Performance for school-aged children and adults with disabilities. *Physical Therapy, 72,* 191–201.

Halom, J. (1991). Assessment of OTA student performance. In *Self-paced instruction for clinical education and supervision* (pp. 287–339). Rockville, MD: American Occupational Therapy Association.

Hamilton, B. B., Granager, C. V., Sherwin, F. S., Zielezny, M., & Tashman, J. S. (1987). A uniform national data system for medical rehabilitation. In M. J. Fuhrer (Ed.), *Rehabilitation outcomes: Analysis and measurement* (pp. 137–146). Baltimore: Paul H. Brookes.

Hubbard, S. (1999). *Occupational therapy attitude scale.* Unpublished manuscript, University of Texas Health Science Center at San Antonio.

Kirchner, G. L., Stone, R. G., & Holm, M. B. (2001). Validation of the fieldwork evaluation for the occupational therapist. *Occupational Therapy in Health Care, 14,* 39–46.

Kolodner, E. L., & Hischmann, C. L. (2000). The role of fieldwork in occupational therapy practice. In S. C. Merrill & P. A. Crist (Eds.), *Meeting the fieldwork challenge: A self-paced clinical course* (pp. 1–20). Bethesda, MD: American Occupational Therapy Association.

Linacre, J. M. (1987–2002). *Many-faceted Rasch measurement computer program.* Chicago: MESA.

Masters, G. N., & Keeves, J. P. (Eds.). (1999). *Advances in measurement in educational research and assessment.* New York: Pergamon.

Mattingly, C. (1991). The narrative nature of clinical reasoning. *American Journal of Occupational Therapy, 45,* 998–1005.

Merbitz, C., Morris, J., & Grip, J. (1989). Ordinal scales and foundations of misinference. *Archives of Physical Medicine and Rehabilitation, 70,* 308–312.

Missiuna, C., Polatajko, H. J., & Ernest-Conibear, M. (1992). Skill acquisition during fieldwork placements in occupational therapy. *Canadian Journal of Occupational Therapy, 59,* 28–39.

National Board for Certification in Occupational Therapy. (1997). *National study for occupational therapy practice* [Executive summary]. Gaithersburg, MD: Author.

Neufeld, V. R., & Norman, G. R. (Eds.). (1985). *Assessing clinical competence.* New York: Springer.

O'Connor, L., & Collier, G. F. (2000). Emerging fieldwork models. In S. C. Merrill & P. A. Crist (Eds.), *Meeting the fieldwork challenge: A self-paced clinical course* (pp. 1–16). Bethesda, MD: American Occupational Therapy Association.

Parham, D. (1987). Toward professionalism: The reflective therapist. *American Journal of Occupational Therapy, 41,* 555–561.

Polatajko, H. J., Lee, L. H., & Bossers, A. M. (1994). Performance evaluation of occupational therapy students: A reliability study. *Canadian Journal of Occupational Therapy, 61,* 20–27.

Rogers, M. W., & Elberth, W. E. (2000). Measuring student fieldwork performance. In S. C. Merrill & P. A. Crist (Eds.), *Meeting the fieldwork challenge: A self-paced clinical course* (pp. 1–52). Bethesda, MD: American Occupational Therapy Association.

Sabari, J. S. (1985). Professional socialization: Implications for occupational therapy education. *American Journal of Occupational Therapy, 39,* 96–102.

Salvatori, P. (1996). Clinical competence: A review of the health care literature with a focus on occupational therapy. *Canadian Journal of Occupational Therapy, 63,* 260–271.

Schell, B. B. (1998). Clinical reasoning: The basis of practice. In M. E. Neistadt & E. B. Crepeau (Eds.), *Willard and Spackman's occupational therapy* (9th ed., pp. 90–100). Philadelphia: Lippincott.

Stutz-Tanenbaum, P., Gaffney, D., Bundy, A., & Fisher, A. G. (1993). *Report of the task force on fieldwork evaluation.* Rockville, MD: American Occupational Therapy Association, Inc.

Townsend, E. (1997). *Enabling occupation: An occupational therapy perspective.* Ottawa: Canadian Association of Occupational Therapy.

van de Vijver, F. J. R. (1986). The robustness of Rasch estimates. *Applied Psychological Measurement, 10,* 45–57.

Velozo, C. A., Kielhofner, G., & Lai, J. S. (1999). The use of Rasch analysis to produce scale-free measurement of functional ability. *American Journal of Occupational Therapy, 53,* 83–90.

Wright, B. D., & Linacre, J. M. (1989). Observations are always ordinal: Measurements, however, must be interval. *Archives of Physical Medicine and Rehabilitation, 70,* 857–860.

Wright, B. D., & Linacre, J. M. (1994). 1994 reasonable mean-square fit values. *Rasch Measurement Transactions, 8,* 370.

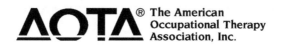® The American
Occupational Therapy
Association, Inc.

Fieldwork Performance Evaluation
For The Occupational Therapy Student

MS./MR.

NAME: (LAST)   (FIRST)   (MIDDLE)

COLLEGE OR UNIVERSITY

FIELDWORK SETTING:

NAME OF ORGANIZATION/FACILITY

ADDRESS: (STREET OR PO BOX)

CITY   STATE   ZIP

TYPE OF FIELDWORK

ORDER OF PLACEMENT 1 2 3 4 OUT OF 1 2 3 4

FROM: TO:
DATES OF PLACEMENT

NUMBER OF HOURS COMPLETED

FINAL SCORE

PASS: _____   **NO PASS:** _____

SIGNATURES:
I HAVE READ THIS REPORT.

SIGNATURE OF STUDENT

NUMBER OF PERSONS CONTRIBUTING TO THIS REPORT

SIGNATURE OF RATER #1

PRINT NAME/CREDENTIALS/POSITION

SIGNATURE OF RATER #2 (IF APPLICABLE)

PRINT NAME/CREDENTIALS/POSITION

SUMMARY COMMENTS:
(ADDRESSES STUDENT'S CLINICAL COMPETENCE)

Fieldwork Performance Evaluation
For The Occupational Therapy Student

This evaluation is a revision of the 1987 American Occupational Therapy Association, Inc. Fieldwork Evaluation Form for the Occupational Therapist and was produced by a committee of the Commission on Education.

PURPOSE

The primary purpose of the Fieldwork Performance Evaluation for the Occupational Therapy Student is to measure entry-level competence of the occupational therapy student. The evaluation is designed to differentiate the competent student from the incompetent student and is not designed to differentiate levels above entry level competence. For further clarification on entry-level competency refer to the Standards of Practice for Occupational Therapy[1].

The evaluation is designed to measure the performance of the occupational therapy process and was not designed to measure the specific occupational therapy tasks in isolation. This evaluation reflects the 1998 Accreditation Council for Occupational Therapy Education Standards[2] and the National Board for Certification in Occupational Therapy, Inc. Practice Analysis results[3]. In addition, this evaluation allows students to evaluate their own strengths and challenges in relation to their performance as an occupational therapist.

USE OF THE FIELDWORK PERFORMANCE EVALUATION FOR THE OCCUPATIONAL THERAPY STUDENT

The Fieldwork Performance Evaluation is intended to provide the student with an accurate assessment of his/her competence for entry-level practice. Both the student and fieldwork educator should recognize that growth occurs over time. **The midterm and final evaluation scores will reflect development of student competency and growth.** In order to effectively use this evaluation to assess student competence, site-specific objectives need to be developed. Utilize this evaluation as a framework to assist in ensuring that all key performance areas are reflected in the site-specific objectives.

Using this evaluation at midterm and final, it is suggested that the student complete a self-evaluation of his/her own performance. During the midterm review process, the student and fieldwork educator should collaboratively develop a plan, which would enable the student to achieve entry-level competence by the end of the fieldwork experience. This plan should include specific objectives and enabling activities to be used by the student and fieldwork educator in order to achieve the desired competence.

The Fieldwork Educator must contact the Academic Fieldwork Coordinator when: (1) a student exhibits unsatisfactory behavior in a substantial number of tasks or (2) a student's potential for achieving entry-level competence by the end of the affiliation is in question.

DIRECTIONS FOR RATING STUDENT PERFORMANCE

- There are 42 performance items.
- Every item must be scored, using the one to four point rating scale (see below).
- **The rating scales should be carefully studied prior to using this evaluation.** Definitions of the scales are given at the top of each page.
- Circle the number that corresponds to the description that best describes the student's performance.
- **The ratings for the Ethics and Safety items must be scored at 3 or above on the final evaluation for the student to pass the fieldwork experience.** If the ratings are below 3, continue to complete the Fieldwork Performance Evaluation to provide feedback to the student on her/his performance.
- Record midterm and final ratings on the Performance Rating Summary Sheet.
- Compare overall midterm and final score to the scale below.

OVERALL MIDTERM SCORE

Satisfactory Performance. . . . . 90 and above
Unsatisfactory Performance. . . . . 89 and below

OVERALL FINAL SCORE

Pass . . . . 122 points and above
No Pass . . . . 121 points and below

RATING SCALE FOR STUDENT PERFORMANCE

4 — **Exceeds Standards:** Performance is highly skilled and self-initiated. This rating is **rarely given** and **would represent the top 5% of all the students** you have supervised.

3 — **Meets Standards:** Performance is consistent with **entry-level** practice. This rating is **infrequently given at midterm** and is a **strong rating at final**.

2 — **Needs improvement:** Performance **is progressing but** still needs improvement for entry-level practice. This is a **realistic rating of performance at midterm**, and some ratings of 2 may be reasonable at the final.

1 — **Unsatisfactory:** Performance is **below standards** and requires development for entry-level practice. This rating is given when **there is a concern about performance.**

RATING SCALE FOR STUDENT PERFORMANCE

4 — **Exceeds Standards:** Performance is highly skilled and self-initiated. This rating is **rarely given** and **would represent the top 5% of all the students** you have supervised.

3 — **Meets Standards:** Performance is consistent with **entry-level** practice. This rating is **infrequently given at midterm** and is a **strong rating at final.**

2 — **Needs improvement:** Performance **is progressing but** still needs improvement for entry-level practice. This is a **realistic rating of performance at midterm,** and some ratings of 2 may be reasonable at the final.

1 — **Unsatisfactory:** Performance is **below standards** and requires development for entry-level practice. This rating is given when **there is a concern about performance.**

I. FUNDAMENTALS OF PRACTICE:

All items in this area must be scored at a #3 or above on the final evaluation in order to pass fieldwork.

1. **Adheres to ethics:** Adheres consistently to the American Occupational Therapy Association Code of Ethics[4] and site's policies and procedures including when relevant, those related to human subject research.

Midterm	1	2	3	4
Final	1	2	3	4

2. **Adheres to safety regulations:** Adheres consistently to safety regulations. Anticipates potentially hazardous situations and takes steps to prevent accidents.

Midterm	1	2	3	4
Final	1	2	3	4

3. **Uses judgment in safety:** Uses sound judgment in regard to safety of self and others during all fieldwork-related activities.

Midterm	1	2	3	4
Final	1	2	3	4

Comments on strengths and areas for improvement:

• **Midterm**

• **Final**

II. BASIC TENETS:

4. Clearly and confidently **articulates the values and beliefs** of the occupational therapy profession to clients, families, significant others, colleagues, service providers, and the public.

Midterm	1	2	3	4
Final	1	2	3	4

5. Clearly, confidently, and accurately **articulates the value of occupation** as a method and desired outcome of occupational therapy to clients, families, significant others, colleagues, service providers, and the public.

Midterm	1	2	3	4
Final	1	2	3	4

6. Clearly, confidently, and accurately **communicates the roles of the occupational therapist and occupational therapy assistant** to clients, families, significant others, colleagues, service providers, and the public.

Midterm	1	2	3	4
Final	1	2	3	4

7. **Collaborates with** client, family, and significant others throughout the occupational therapy process.

Midterm	1	2	3	4
Final	1	2	3	4

Comments on strengths and areas for improvement:

• **Midterm**

RATING SCALE FOR STUDENT PERFORMANCE

4 — **Exceeds Standards:** Performance is highly skilled and self-initiated. This rating is **rarely given** and **would represent the top 5% of all the students** you have supervised.

3 — **Meets Standards:** Performance is consistent with **entry-level** practice. This rating is **infrequently given at midterm** and is a **strong rating at final**.

2 — **Needs improvement:** Performance **is progressing but** still needs improvement for entry-level practice. This is a **realistic rating of performance at midterm**, and some ratings of 2 may be reasonable at the final.

1 — **Unsatisfactory:** Performance is **below standards** and requires development for entry-level practice. This rating is given when **there is a concern about performance.**

III. EVALUATION AND SCREENING:

8. **Articulates a clear and logical rationale** for the evaluation process.

Midterm	1	2	3	4
Final	1	2	3	4

9. **Selects relevant screening and assessment methods** while considering such factors as client's priorities, context(s), theories, and evidence-based practice.

Midterm	1	2	3	4
Final	1	2	3	4

10. **Determines client's occupational profile** and performance through appropriate assessment methods.

Midterm	1	2	3	4
Final	1	2	3	4

11. **Assesses client factors and context(s)** that support or hinder occupational performance.

Midterm	1	2	3	4
Final	1	2	3	4

12. **Obtains sufficient and necessary information** from relevant resources such as client, families, significant others, service providers, and records prior to and during the evaluation process.

Midterm	1	2	3	4
Final	1	2	3	4

13. **Administers assessments** in a uniform manner to ensure findings are valid and reliable.

Midterm	1	2	3	4
Final	1	2	3	4

14. **Adjusts/modifies the assessment procedures** based on client's needs, behaviors, and culture.

Midterm	1	2	3	4
Final	1	2	3	4

15. **Interprets evaluation results** to determine client's occupational performance strengths and challenges.

Midterm	1	2	3	4
Final	1	2	3	4

16. **Establishes an accurate and appropriate plan** based on the evaluation results, through integrating multiple factors such as client's priorities, context(s), theories, and evidence-based practice.

Midterm	1	2	3	4
Final	1	2	3	4

17. **Documents the results of the evaluation** process that demonstrates objective measurement of client's occupational performance.

Midterm	1	2	3	4
Final	1	2	3	4

Comments on strengths and areas for improvement:

• **Midterm**

• **Final**

IV. INTERVENTION:

18. **Articulates a clear and logical rationale** for the intervention process.

Midterm	1	2	3	4
Final	1	2	3	4

19. **Utilizes evidence** from published research and relevant resources to make informed intervention decisions.

Midterm	1	2	3	4
Final	1	2	3	4

20. **Chooses occupations** that motivate and challenge clients.

Midterm	1	2	3	4
Final	1	2	3	4

21. **Selects relevant occupations** to facilitate clients meeting established goals.

Midterm	1	2	3	4
Final	1	2	3	4

22. **Implements intervention plans that are client-centered.**

Midterm	1	2	3	4
Final	1	2	3	4

23. **Implements intervention plans that are occupation-based.**

Midterm	1	2	3	4
Final	1	2	3	4

24. **Modifies task approach, occupations, and the environment** to maximize client performance.

Midterm	1	2	3	4
Final	1	2	3	4

25. **Updates, modifies, or terminates the intervention plan** based upon careful monitoring of the client's status.

Midterm	1	2	3	4
Final	1	2	3	4

26. **Documents client's response** to services in a manner that demonstrates the efficacy of interventions.

Midterm	1	2	3	4
Final	1	2	3	4

Comments on strengths and areas for improvement:

• **Midterm**

• **Final**

V. MANAGEMENT OF OCCUPATIONAL THERAPY SERVICES:

27. **Demonstrates through practice or discussion the ability to assign** appropriate responsibilities to the occupational therapy assistant and occupational therapy aide.

Midterm	1	2	3	4
Final	1	2	3	4

28. **Demonstrates through practice or discussion the ability to actively collaborate** with the occupational therapy assistant.

Midterm	1	2	3	4
Final	1	2	3	4

29. **Demonstrates understanding of the costs and funding** related to occupational therapy services at this site.

Midterm	1	2	3	4
Final	1	2	3	4

30. **Accomplishes organizational goals** by establishing priorities, developing strategies, and meeting deadlines.

Midterm	1	2	3	4
Final	1	2	3	4

31. **Produces the volume of work** required in the expected time frame.

Midterm	1	2	3	4
Final	1	2	3	4

Comments on strengths and areas for improvement:

• **Midterm**

• **Final**

SAMPLE

SAMPLE

RATING SCALE FOR STUDENT PERFORMANCE

4 — **Exceeds Standards:** Performance is highly skilled and self-initiated. This rating is **rarely given** and **would represent the top 5% of all the students** you have supervised.

3 — **Meets Standards:** Performance is consistent with **entry-level** practice. This rating is **infrequently given at midterm** and is a **strong rating at final.**

2 — **Needs improvement:** Performance **is progressing but** still needs improvement for entry-level practice. This is a **realistic rating of performance at midterm**, and some ratings of 2 may be reasonable at the final.

1 — **Unsatisfactory:** Performance is **below standards** and requires development for entry-level practice. This rating is given when **there is a concern about performance.**

VI. COMMUNICATION:

32. **Clearly and effectively communicates verbally and nonverbally** with clients, families, significant others, colleagues, service providers, and the public.

Midterm	1	2	3	4
Final	1	2	3	4

33. **Produces clear and accurate documentation** according to site requirements.

Midterm	1	2	3	4
Final	1	2	3	4

34. **All written communication is legible,** using proper spelling, punctuation, and grammar.

Midterm	1	2	3	4
Final	1	2	3	4

35. **Uses language appropriate to the recipient** of the information, including but not limited to funding agencies and regulatory agencies.

Midterm	1	2	3	4
Final	1	2	3	4

Comments on strengths and areas for improvement:

• **Midterm**

• **Final**

VII. PROFESSIONAL BEHAVIORS:

36. **Collaborates with supervisor(s)** to maximize the learning experience.

Midterm	1	2	3	4
Final	1	2	3	4

37. **Takes responsibility for attaining professional competence** by seeking out learning opportunities and interactions with supervisor(s) and others.

Midterm	1	2	3	4
Final	1	2	3	4

38. **Responds constructively to feedback.**

Midterm	1	2	3	4
Final	1	2	3	4

39. **Demonstrates consistent work behaviors** including initiative, preparedness, dependability, and work site maintenance.

Midterm	1	2	3	4
Final	1	2	3	4

40. **Demonstrates effective time management.**

Midterm	1	2	3	4
Final	1	2	3	4

41. **Demonstrates positive interpersonal skills** including but not limited to cooperation, flexibility, tact, and empathy.

Midterm	1	2	3	4
Final	1	2	3	4

42. **Demonstrates respect for diversity** factors of others including but not limited to socio-cultural, socioeconomic, spiritual, and lifestyle choices.

Midterm	1	2	3	4
Final	1	2	3	4

Comments on strengths and areas for improvement:

• **Midterm**

• **Final**

PERFORMANCE RATING SUMMARY SHEET

Performance Items	Midterm Ratings	Final Ratings
I. FUNDAMENTALS OF PRACTICE		
1. Adheres to ethics		
2. Adheres to safety regulations		
3. Uses judgment in safety		
II. BASIC TENETS OF OCCUPATIONAL THERAPY		
4. Articulates values and beliefs		
5. Articulates value of occupation		
6. Communicates role of occupational therapist		
7. Collaborates with clients		
III. EVALUATION AND SCREENING		
8. Articulates clear rationale for evaluation		
9. Selects relevant methods		
10. Determines occupational profile		
11. Assesses client and contextual factors		
12. Obtains sufficient and necessary information		
13. Administers assessments		
14. Adjusts/modifies assessment procedures		
15. Interprets evaluation results		
16. Establishes accurate plan		
17. Documents results of evaluation		
IV. INTERVENTION		
18. Articulates clear rationale for intervention		
19. Utilizes evidence to make informed decisions		
20. Chooses occupations that motivate and challenge		
21. Selects relevant occupations		
22. Implements client-centered interventions		
23. Implements occupation-based interventions		
24. Modifies approach, occupation, and environment		
25. Updates, modifies, or terminates intervention plan		
26. Documents client's response		
V. MANAGEMENT OF OT SERVICES		
27. Demonstrates ability to assign through practice or discussion		
28. Demonstrates ability to collaborate through practice or discussion		
29. Understands costs and funding		
30. Accomplishes organizational goals		
31. Produces work in expected time frame		
VI. COMMUNICATION		
32. Communicates verbally and nonverbally		
33. Produces clear documentation		
34. Written communication is legible		
35. Uses language appropriate to recipient		
VII. PROFESSIONAL BEHAVIORS		
36. Collaborates with supervisor		
37. Takes responsibility for professional competence		
38. Responds constructively to feedback		
39. Demonstrates consistent work behaviors		
40. Demonstrates time management		
41. Demonstrates positive interpersonal skills		
42. Demonstrates respect for diversity		
TOTAL SCORE		

MIDTERM:

Satisfactory Performance . . . . 90 and above

Unsatisfactory Performance . . . . 89 and below

FINAL:

Pass . . . . 122 points and above

No Pass . . . . 121 points and below

REFERENCES

1. American Occupational Therapy Association. (1998). Standards of practice for occupational therapy. *American Journal of Occupational Therapy, 52,* 866–869.
2. Accreditation Council for Occupational Therapy Education. (1999). Standards for an accredited educational program for the occupational therapist. *American Journal of Occupational Therapy, 53,* 575–582.
3. National Board for Certification in Occupational Therapy. (1997). *National Study of Occupational Therapy Practice, Executive Summary.*
4. American Occupational Therapy Association. (2000). Occupational therapy code of ethics (2000). *American Journal of Occupational Therapy, 54,* 614–616.
5. American Occupational Therapy Association (2002). Occupational therapy practice framework: Domain and process. *American Journal of Occupational Therapy, 56,* 606–639.

GLOSSARY

Client Factors: Those factors that reside within the client and that may affect performance in areas of occupation. Client factors include body functions and body structures
• body functions (a client factor, including physical, cognitive, psychosocial aspects)—"the physiological function of body systems (including psychological functions)" (WHO, 2001, p.10)
• body structures—"anatomical parts of the body such as organs, limbs and their components [that support body function]" (WHO, 2001, p.10)
(Occupational therapy practice framework: Domain and process. *American Journal of Occupational Therapy, 56,* 606–639.)[5]

Code of Ethics: Refer to www.aota.org/general/coe.asp

Collaborate: To work together with a mutual sharing of thoughts and ideas (ACOTE Glossary)

Competency: Adequate skills and abilities to practice as an entry-level occupational therapist or occupational therapy assistant

Context: Refers to a variety of interrelated conditions within and surrounding the client that influence performance. Contexts include cultural, physical, social, personal, spiritual, temporal and virtual. (Occupational therapy practice framework: Domain and process. *American Journal of Occupational Therapy, 56,* 606–639)[5]

Efficacy: Having the desired influence or outcome (from Neistadt and Crepeau, eds. *Willard & Spackman's Occupational Therapy,* 9th edition, 1998)

Entry-level practice: Refer to American Occupational Therapy Association (1993). Occupational therapy roles. *American Journal of Occupational Therapy, 47,* 1087–99.

Evidence-based Practice: "Conscientious, explicit and judicious use of current best evidence in making decisions about the care of individual patients. The practice of evidence-based [health care] means integrating individual clinical expertise with the best available external clinical evidence from systematic research." (Sackett and colleagues, Evidence-based medicine: How to practice and teach EBM, 1997, p. 2) (*From the Mary Law article "Evidence-Based Practice: What Can It Mean for ME?",* www.aota.org)

Occupation: Groups of activities and tasks of everyday life, named, organized, and given value and meaning by individuals and a culture; occupation is everything people do to occupy themselves, including looking after themselves (self-care), enjoying life (leisure), and contributing to the social and economic fabric of their communities (productivity); the domain of concern and the therapeutic medium of occupational therapy. (Townsend, ed., 1997, *Enabling Occupation: An Occupational Therapy Perspective,* p.181)

Occupational Performance: The result of a dynamic, interwoven relationship between persons, environment, and occupation over a person's lifespan; the ability to choose, organize, and satisfactorily perform meaningful occupations that are culturally defined and age appropriate for looking after oneself, enjoying life, and contributing to the social and economic fabric of a community. (Townsend, ed., 1997, *Enabling Occupation: An Occupational Therapy Perspective,* p.181)

Occupational Profile: A profile that describes the client's occupational history, patterns of daily living, interests, values and needs. (Occupational therapy practice framework: Domain and process. *American Journal of Occupational Therapy, 56,* 606–639)[5]

Spiritual: (a context) The fundamental orientation of a person's life; that which inspires and motivates that individual. (Occupational therapy practice framework: Domain and process. *American Journal of Occupational Therapy, 56,* 606–639)[5]

Theory: "An organized way of thinking about given phenomena. In occupational therapy the phenomenon of concern is occupational endeavor. Theory attempts to (1) define and explain the relationships between concepts or ideas related to the phenomenon of interest, (2) explain how these relationships can predict behavior or events, and (3) suggest ways that the phenomenon can be changed or controlled. Occupational therapy theory is concerned with four major concepts related to occupational endeavor: person, environment, health, and occupation." (Neistadt and Crepeau, eds., *Willard & Spackman's Occupational Therapy,* 9th ed., 1998, p. 521)

© 2002 by the American Occupational Therapy Association, Inc. All rights reserved.

No part of this evaluation may be reproduced in whole or in part by any means without permission.

Printed in the United States of America.

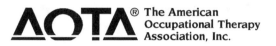

Fieldwork Performance Evaluation
For The Occupational Therapy Assistant Student

MS./MR.
_____

NAME: (LAST)   (FIRST)   (MIDDLE)

_____

COLLEGE OR UNIVERSITY

FIELDWORK SETTING:

_____

NAME OF ORGANIZATION/FACILITY

_____

ADDRESS: (STREET OR PO BOX)

_____

CITY   STATE   ZIP

_____

TYPE OF FIELDWORK

ORDER OF PLACEMENT: 1 2 3 4   OUT OF 1 2 3 4

FROM: _____ TO: _____

DATES OF PLACEMENT

_____

NUMBER OF HOURS COMPLETED

FINAL SCORE

PASS: _____   NO PASS: _____

SIGNATURES:

I HAVE READ THIS REPORT.

_____

SIGNATURE OF STUDENT

_____

NUMBER OF PERSONS CONTRIBUTING TO THIS REPORT

_____

SIGNATURE OF RATER #1

_____

PRINT NAME/CREDENTIALS/POSITION

_____

SIGNATURE OF RATER #2 (IF APPLICABLE)

_____

PRINT NAME/CREDENTIALS/POSITION

SUMMARY COMMENTS:
(ADDRESSES STUDENT'S CLINICAL COMPETENCE)

Fieldwork Performance Evaluation
For The Occupational Therapy Assistant Student

This evaluation is a revision of the 1983 American Occupational Therapy Association, Inc. Fieldwork Evaluation Form for the Occupational Therapy Assistant and was produced by a committee of the Commission on Education.

PURPOSE

The primary purpose of the Fieldwork Performance Evaluation for the Occupational Therapy Assistant Student is to measure entry-level competence of the occupational therapy assistant student. The evaluation is designed to differentiate the competent student from the incompetent student and is not designed to differentiate levels above entry level competence. For further clarification on entry-level competency refer to the Standards of Practice for Occupational Therapy[1].

The evaluation is designed to measure the performance of the occupational therapy process and was not designed to measure the specific occupational therapy tasks in isolation. This evaluation reflects the 1998 Accreditation Council for Occupational Therapy Education Standards[2] and the National Board for Certification in Occupational Therapy, Inc. Practice Analysis results[3]. In addition, this evaluation allows students to evaluate their own strengths and challenges in relation to their performance as an occupational therapy assistant.

USE OF THE FIELDWORK PERFORMANCE EVALUATION FOR THE OCCUPATIONAL THERAPY STUDENT

The Fieldwork Performance Evaluation is intended to provide the student with an accurate assessment of his/her competence for entry-level practice. Both the student and fieldwork educator should recognize that growth occurs over time. **The midterm and final evaluation scores will reflect development of student competency and growth.** In order to effectively use this evaluation to assess student competence, site-specific objectives need to be developed. Utilize this evaluation as a framework to assist in ensuring that all key performance areas are reflected in the site-specific objectives.

Using this evaluation at midterm and final, it is suggested that the student complete a self-evaluation of his/her own performance. During the midterm review process, the student and fieldwork educator should collaboratively develop a plan, which would enable the student to achieve entry-level competence by the end of the fieldwork experience. This plan should include specific objectives and enabling activities to be used by the student and fieldwork educator in order to achieve the desired competence.

The Fieldwork Educator must contact the Academic Fieldwork Coordinator when: (1) a student exhibits unsatisfactory behavior in a substantial number of tasks or (2) a student's potential for achieving entry-level competence by the end of the affiliation is in question.

DIRECTIONS FOR RATING STUDENT PERFORMANCE

- There are 25 performance items.
- Every item must be scored, using the one to four point rating scale (see below).
- **The rating scales should be carefully studied prior to using this evaluation.** Definitions of the scales are given at the top of each page.
- Circle the number that corresponds to the description that best describes the student's performance.
- **The ratings for the Ethics and Safety items must be scored at 3 or above on the final evaluation for the student to pass the fieldwork experience.** If the ratings are below 3, continue to complete the Fieldwork Performance Evaluation to provide feedback to the student on her/his performance.
- Record midterm and final ratings on the Performance Rating Summary Sheet.
- Compare overall midterm and final score to the scale below.

OVERALL MIDTERM SCORE

Satisfactory Performance . . . . 54 and above
Unsatisfactory Performance . . . . 53 and below

OVERALL FINAL SCORE

Pass . . . . 70 points and above
No Pass . . . . 69 points and below

RATING SCALE FOR STUDENT PERFORMANCE

4 — **Exceeds Standards:** Performance is highly skilled and self-initiated. This rating is **rarely given** and **would represent the top 5% of all the students** you have supervised.

3 — **Meets Standards:** Performance is consistent with **entry-level** practice. This rating is **infrequently given at midterm** and is a **strong rating at final**.

2 — **Needs improvement:** Performance **is progressing but** still needs improvement for entry-level practice. This is a **realistic rating of performance at midterm**, and some ratings of 2 may be reasonable at the final.

1 — **Unsatisfactory:** Performance is **below standards** and requires development for entry-level practice. This rating is given when **there is a concern about performance**.

RATING SCALE FOR STUDENT PERFORMANCE

4 — **Exceeds Standards:** Performance is highly skilled and self-initiated. This rating is **rarely given** and **would represent the top 5% of all the students** you have supervised.

3 — **Meets Standards:** Performance is consistent with **entry-level** practice. This rating is **infrequently given at midterm** and is a **strong rating at final.**

2 — **Needs improvement:** Performance **is progressing but** still needs improvement for entry-level practice. This is a **realistic rating of performance at midterm**, and some ratings of 2 may be reasonable at the final.

1 — **Unsatisfactory:** Performance is **below standards** and requires development for entry-level practice. This rating is given when **there is a concern about performance.**

I. FUNDAMENTALS OF PRACTICE:

All items in this area must be scored at a #3 or above on the final evaluation in order to pass fieldwork.

1. **Ethics:** Adheres consistently to the American Occupational Therapy Association Code of Ethics[4] and site's policies and procedures.

Midterm	1	2	3	4
Final	1	2	3	4

2. **Safety:** Adheres consistently to safety regulations. Anticipates potentially hazardous situations and takes steps to prevent accidents.

Midterm	1	2	3	4
Final	1	2	3	4

3. **Safety:** Uses sound judgment in regard to safety of self and others during all fieldwork-related activities.

Midterm	1	2	3	4
Final	1	2	3	4

Comments on strengths and areas for improvement

- **Midterm**

- **Final**

II. BASIC TENETS OF OCCUPATIONAL THERAPY

4. **Occupational Therapy Philosophy:** Clearly communicates the values and beliefs of occupational therapy, highlighting the use of occupation to clients, families, significant others, and service providers.

Midterm	1	2	3	4
Final	1	2	3	4

5. **Occupational Therapist/Occupational Therapy Assistant Roles:** Communicates the roles of the occupational therapist and occupational therapy assistant to clients, families, significant others, and service providers.

Midterm	1	2	3	4
Final	1	2	3	4

6. **Evidenced-based Practice:** Makes informed practice decisions based on published research and relevant informational resources.

Midterm	1	2	3	4
Final	1	2	3	4

Comments on strengths and areas for improvement

- **Midterm**

- **Final**

RATING SCALE FOR STUDENT PERFORMANCE

4 — **Exceeds Standards:** Performance is highly skilled and self-initiated. This rating is **rarely given** and **would represent the top 5% of all the students** you have supervised.

3 — **Meets Standards:** Performance is consistent with **entry-level** practice. This rating is **infrequently given at midterm** and is a **strong rating at final**.

2 — **Needs improvement:** Performance **is progressing but** still needs improvement for entry-level practice. This is a **realistic rating of performance at midterm**, and some ratings of 2 may be reasonable at the final.

1 — **Unsatisfactory:** Performance is **below standards** and requires development for entry-level practice. This rating is given when **there is a concern about performance**.

III. EVALUATION/SCREENING:

(Includes daily evaluation of interventions)

7. **Gathers Data:** Under the supervision of and in cooperation with the occupational therapist and/or occupational therapy assistant, accurately gathers relevant information regarding a client's occupations of self care, productivity, leisure, and the factors that support and hinder occupational performance.

Midterm	1	2	3	4
Final	1	2	3	4

8. **Administers Assessments:** Establishes service competency in assessment methods, including but not limited to interviews, observations, assessment tools, and chart reviews within the context of the service delivery setting.

Midterm	1	2	3	4
Final	1	2	3	4

9. **Interprets:** Assists with interpreting assessments in relation to the client's performance and goals in collaboration with the occupational therapist.

Midterm	1	2	3	4
Final	1	2	3	4

10. **Reports:** Reports results accurately in a clear, concise manner that reflects the client's status and goals.

Midterm	1	2	3	4
Final	1	2	3	4

11. **Establish Goals:** Develops client-centered and occupation-based goals in collaboration with the occupational therapist.

Midterm	1	2	3	4
Final	1	2	3	4

Comments on strengths and areas for improvement

- Midterm

- Final

IV. INTERVENTION:

12. **Plans Intervention:** In collaboration with the occupational therapist, establishes methods, duration, and frequency of interventions that are client-centered and occupation-based. Intervention plans reflect context of setting.

Midterm	1	2	3	4
Final	1	2	3	4

13. **Selects Intervention:** Selects and sequences relevant interventions that promote the client's ability to engage in occupations.

Midterm	1	2	3	4
Final	1	2	3	4

14. **Implements Intervention:** Implements occupation-based interventions effectively in collaboration with clients, families, significant others, and service providers.

Midterm	1	2	3	4
Final	1	2	3	4

SAMPLE

15. **Activity Analysis:** Grades activities to motivate and challenge clients in order to facilitate progress.

Midterm	1	2	3	4
Final	1	2	3	4

16. **Therapeutic Use of Self:** Effectively interacts with clients to facilitate accomplishment of established goals.

Midterm	1	2	3	4
Final	1	2	3	4

17. **Modifies Intervention Plan:** Monitors the client's status in order to update, change, or terminate the intervention plan in collaboration with the occupational therapist.

Midterm	1	2	3	4
Final	1	2	3	4

Comments on strengths and areas for improvement

• Midterm

• Final

V. COMMUNICATION:

18. **Verbal/Nonverbal Communication:** Clearly and effectively communicates verbally and nonverbally with clients, families, significant others, colleagues, service providers, and the public.

Midterm	1	2	3	4
Final	1	2	3	4

19. **Written Communication:** Produces clear and accurate documentation according to site requirements. All writing is legible, using proper spelling, punctuation, and grammar.

Midterm	1	2	3	4
Final	1	2	3	4

Comments on strengths and areas for improvement

• Midterm

• Final

RATING SCALE FOR STUDENT PERFORMANCE

4 — **Exceeds Standards:** Performance is highly skilled and self-initiated. This rating is **rarely given** and **would represent the top 5% of all the students** you have supervised.

3 — **Meets Standards:** Performance is consistent with **entry-level** practice. This rating is **infrequently given at midterm** and is a **strong rating at final**.

2 — **Needs improvement:** Performance **is progressing but** still needs improvement for entry-level practice. This is a **realistic rating of performance at midterm**, and some ratings of 2 may be reasonable at the final.

1 — **Unsatisfactory:** Performance is **below standards** and requires development for entry-level practice. This rating is given when **there is a concern about performance**.

VI. PROFESSIONAL BEHAVIORS:

20. **Self-Responsibility:** Takes responsibility for attaining professional competence by seeking out learning opportunities and interactions with supervisor(s) and others.

Midterm	1	2	3	4
Final	1	2	3	4

21. **Responds to Feedback:** Responds constructively to feedback.

Midterm	1	2	3	4
Final	1	2	3	4

22. **Work Behaviors:** Demonstrates consistent work behaviors including initiative, preparedness, dependability, and work site maintenance.

Midterm	1	2	3	4
Final	1	2	3	4

23. **Time Management:** Demonstrates effective time management.

Midterm	1	2	3	4
Final	1	2	3	4

24. **Interpersonal Skills:** Demonstrates positive interpersonal skills including but not limited to cooperation, flexibility, tact, and empathy.

Midterm	1	2	3	4
Final	1	2	3	4

25. **Cultural Competence:** Demonstrates respect for diversity factors of others including but not limited to sociocultural, socioeconomic, spiritual, and lifestyle choices.

Midterm	1	2	3	4
Final	1	2	3	4

Comments on strengths and areas for improvement

• Midterm

• Final

PERFORMANCE RATING SUMMARY SHEET

Performance Items	Midterm Ratings	Final Ratings
I. FUNDAMENTALS OF PRACTICE		
1. Ethics		
2. Safety (adheres)		
3. Safety (judgment)		
II. BASIC TENETS OF OCCUPATIONAL THERAPY		
4. OT philosophy		
5. OT/OTA roles		
6. Evidenced-based practice		
III. EVALUATION/SCREENING (includes daily evaluation of interventions)		
7. Gathers data		
8. Administers assessments		
9. Interprets		
10. Reports		
11. Establishes goals		
IV. INTERVENTION		
12. Plans intervention		
13. Selects intervention		
14. Implements intervention		
15. Activity analysis		
16. Therapeutic use of self		
17. Modifies intervention plan		
V. COMMUNICATION		
18. Verbal/nonverbal communication		
19. Written communication		
VI. PROFESSIONAL BEHAVIORS		
20. Self-responsibility		
21. Responds to feedback		
22. Work behaviors		
23. Time management		
24. Interpersonal skills		
25. Cultural competence		
TOTAL SCORE		

MIDTERM:

Satisfactory Performance. . . . . 54 and above

Unsatisfactory Performance. . . . . 53 and below

FINAL:

Pass . . . . 70 points and above

No Pass . . . . 69 points and below

REFERENCES

1. American Occupational Therapy Association. (1998). Standards of practice for occupational therapy. *American Journal of Occupational Therapy, 52,* 866–869.
2. Accreditation Council for Occupational Therapy Education. (1999). Standards for an accredited educational program for the occupational therapy assistant. *American Journal of Occupational Therapy, 53,* 583–589.
3. National Board for Certification in Occupational Therapy. (1997). *National Study of Occupational Therapy Practice, Executive Summary.*
4. American Occupational Therapy Association. (2000). Occupational therapy code of ethics (2000). *American Journal of Occupational Therapy, 54,* 614–616.
5. American Occupational Therapy Association (2002). Occupational therapy practice framework: Domain and process. *American Journal of Occupational Therapy, 56,* 606–639.

GLOSSARY

Activity Analysis: "A way of thinking used to understand activities, the performance components to do them and the cultural meanings typically ascribed to them" (Neistadt and Crepeau, 1998, *Willard and Spackman's Occupational Therapy,* 9th ed., p. 135)

Code of Ethics: Refer to www.aota.org/general/coe.asp

Collaborate: To work together with a mutual sharing of thoughts and ideas (ACOTE Glossary)

Competency: Adequate skills and abilities to practice as an entry-level occupational therapist or occupational therapy assistant

Entry-level practice: Refer to American Occupational Therapy Association. (1993). Occupational therapy roles. *American Journal of Occupational Therapy, 47,* 1087–99.

Evidence-based Practice: "Conscientious, explicit, and judicious use of current best evidence in making decisions about the care of individual patients. The practice of evidence-based [health care] means integrating individual clinical expertise with the best available external clinical evidence from systematic research." (Sackett and colleagues, Evidence-based medicine: How to practice and teach EBM, 1997, p. 2) (*From the Mary Law article "Evidence-Based Practice: What Can It Mean for ME?",* www.aota.org)

Occupation: Groups of activities and tasks of everyday life, named, organized, and given value and meaning by individuals and a culture; occupation is everything people do to occupy themselves, including looking after themselves (self-care), enjoying life (leisure), and contributing to the social and economic fabric of their communities (productivity); the domain of concern and the therapeutic medium of occupational therapy. (Townsend, ed., 1997, *Enabling Occupation: An Occupational Therapy Perspective,* p.181)

Occupational Performance: The result of a dynamic, interwoven relationship between persons, environment, and occupation over a person's life span; the ability to choose, organize, and satisfactorily perform meaningful occupations that are culturally defined and age appropriate for looking after oneself, enjoying life, and contributing to the social and economic fabric of a community. (Townsend, ed., 1997, *Enabling Occupation: An Occupational Therapy Perspective,* p.181)

Spiritual: (a context) The fundamental orientation of a person's life; that which inspires and motivates that individual. (Occupational therapy practice framework: Domain and process. *American Journal of Occupational Therapy, 56,* 606–639)[5]

© 2002 by the American Occupational Therapy Association, Inc. All rights reserved.

No part of this evaluation may be reproduced in whole or in part by any means without permission.

Printed in the United States of America.

About the Author

KAREN ATLER, MS, OTR, is an assistant professor in the Occupational Therapy Department at Colorado State University, Fort Collins. She served as cochair of the Fieldwork Evaluation Revision Task Force from 1998 to 2002. She has been involved in fieldwork education for most of her 22 years as an occupational therapist, both as a practitioner and an educator. Karen participated in the American Occupational Therapy Foundation grant related to fieldwork that resulted in the development of the Fieldwork Experience Assessment Tool, coordinated and developed Level I fieldwork sites, and has supervised both Level I and Level II fieldwork students in emerging practice areas.